Ethics, Injuries and the Law in $

For all who believe
in
The Corinthian Ideal
of
Fair Play and the Rule of Law
In Sport, and Society, too

# Ethics, Injuries and the Law in Sports Medicine

Edward Grayson MA (Oxon)

*Barrister of the Middle Temple and of the South Eastern Circuit;*
*Visiting Professor of Sport and the Law in the Anglia Law School,*
*Anglia Polytechnic University;*
*Founding President, British Association for Sport and the Law;*
*Fellow of the Royal Society of Medicine*

With forewords by

Dr Delon Human MB, ChB, MFGP, M.Prix.Med, DCH
*Secretary General, World Medical Association Inc.*

and

Professor Donald Macleod MB, ChB, FRCSEd, FRCPEd, DipSpMed
*Honorary Professor of Sports Medicine (Aberdeen University);*
*Chairman, Intercollegiate Academic Board of Sports and Exercise Medicine;*
*President, British Association of Sport and Medicine;*
*Honorary Medical Adviser, Scottish Rugby Union and*
*Member of the International Rugby Board Medical Advisory Committee*

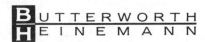

OXFORD AUCKLAND BOSTON JOHANNESBURG MELBOURNE NEW DELHI

Butterworth-Heinemann
Linacre House, Jordan Hill, Oxford OX2 8DP
225 Wildwood Avenue, Woburn, MA 01801-2041
A division of Reed Educational and Professional Publishing Ltd

℞ A member of the Reed Elsevier plc group

First published 1999

**British Library Cataloguing in Publication Data**
Grayson, Edward
  Ethics, injuries and the law in sports medicine
  1.  Sports medicine     2.  Sports medicine – Law and legislation
  3.  Medical ethics
  I.  Title
  617.1′027

ISBN 0 7506 1576 1

Data manipulation by David Gregson Associates, Beccles, Suffolk
Printed and bound in Great Britain by Biddles Ltd, Guildford and Kings Lynn

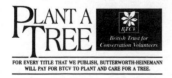

# Contents

'... aversion to law and courts of law
is naturally strong in the human mind.'

Lord Hewart, The Lord Chief Justice of England
*Introduction to Uncommon Law*
by A. P. Herbert (1935)

# Foreword I  by Dr Delon Human

At a time when the grave dangers of doping and violence in sport, and those participating in the process are becoming more apparent, the timing of this book could not have been better planned. There is a crying need for guidance by not only physicians, sports administrators, jurists, and the governmental and commercial sectors, but most of all by athletes, and the spectators who enjoy watching sport.

Professor Grayson's book offers just the kind of leadership which is necessary at this stage. It is a lucid, comprehensive and compelling exposition of guidelines that should be applied to protect athletes at both competitively professional and recreational levels, and safeguard sport as an international treasure.

It is significant that Professor Grayson regards the world's physicians as key players in this complex situation. The World Medical Association (WMA), the global representative body of physicians, has set up guidelines for physicians involved in sports medicine, which are brilliantly described in this book. However, in professional sport it is now known that all physicians do not follow these guidelines In exceptional cases, some physicians have overstepped the line of professional ethics, and have become involved in 'managing', and even concealment of doping in sport. This is contrary to the profession's code of conduct, and definitely not in the best interests of their patients. Here Professor Grayson makes an important contribution to the ethical framework that should be followed by all involved in sport

On graduating as physicians, an oath is usually made – 'the health of my patient will be my first consideration'. Professor Grayson urges the world community to apply this principle in considering first the health and safety of our athletes who participate in the widely contrasting and differing professional and recreational fields of play. We thank him for this insight, and for an outstanding contribution to world sport, medicine and the law.

17 March, 1999

# Foreword II   by Professor Donald Macleod

Exercise and temperance can preserve something of our early strength, even in old age.

(Cicero 106–43 BC)

The wisdom of Cicero's advice to the citizens of Rome has been lost to us for the best part of two millennia. It is a recent development that regular exercise has been accepted by the medical profession as well as the Public Health Services and Government as one of the essential socio-economic components required to maintain a normal, healthy and active lifestyle. The teaching profession is also reviewing and renewing the role of sport and exercise in education.

Participation in regular exercise, appropriate for the individual, should be free of all reasonable risks if it is to benefit health. Regular exercise has also been convincingly demonstrated to be an essential component for successful rehabilitation following a wide range of illnesses, injuries and operations.

In an ideal world, regular exercise would be built into the lifestyle of the very young and continued throughout youth into maturity and later life. The patterns of exercise may vary with ageing but the habit of regular exercise should be continued principally to help the cardiovascular, metabolic, respiratory and loco-motor systems – to maintain physical and psychological self-sufficiency into old age.

Accordingly, any individual can reasonably expect their medical adviser to clearly understand the role of regular exercise in health promotion as well as the management of disease or disability. I do not believe that medicine and its allied professions can avoid this responsibility and Professor Grayson has highlighted this point in his text.

The main theme of *Ethics, Injuries and the Law in Sports Medicine* relates to sport more than exercise. Sport invariably carries risk. Sport implies competition – against oneself, the stopwatch, other participants and teams, or the environment and elements. Successes in sport are achieved by appropriate preparation in conjunction with a calculation of the risks involved including injury, illness or even death. Participation in a sport implies that the participants are aware of and accept the legitimate risks inherent in that sport.

Doctors and allied professionals in a wide range of clinical practice including primary care, hospital based specialists and the community will regularly encounter sports participants. These patients can reasonably expect to receive competent professional advice regarding their injury or illness and how it will affect the sporting aspect of their lifestyle. 'Give it up' is not longer acceptable to the general public.

Doctors and allied professionals who choose to become involved in sport, whether on a voluntary, 'in kind' or paid basis must recognize that their commitment is welcomed because of their professional expertise. The club, its members and its officials can justifiably expect clinical competence plus a little more – an additional skill when dealing with their sport and its participants. The medical team supporting a sport needs to be able to demonstrate appropriate qualifications, experience and continuing medical education and professional development in their respective speciality – medicine, physiotherapy, nutrition, psychology etc. If you, as a doctor, or member of the professions allied to medicine, are not convinced of the truth of these proposals – then reading Professor Grayson's text will emphasize the point. Sports participants are not above the law and they are not second-class patients. Carefully planned, evidence based, audited and documented clinical practice is just as important at the touchline, in the swimming pool, in the gymnasium, or at the horse or motor racing circuit as it is in the consulting room.

Elite and professional sport are facing a crisis with loss of public confidence in activities and participants who were, until the recent past, looked on as national role models for the young and unifying forces in society.

Drugs, corruption by outside influences and cheating by individuals, greed driving exorbitant wage packets and transfer fees, condoned violence increasing injuries as well as perceived exploitation of spectators and TV audiences paint a very unhappy picture. Sport is increasingly seen to be under the control of inappropriate and unrelated outside influences such as the media and commerce through sponsorship and advertising.

Medicine and its allied professions are not without blame in the this unsavoury and depressing picture – particularly with regard to problems with drug use and abuse and the prevention of injuries. The medical professions can make a positive contribution to sport and this has been highlighted by Professor Grayson in his text by discussing and expanding the World Medical Association Guidelines on Sport, reminding us all of our ethical duties to individual patients as well as society by drawing our attention to relevant aspects of legal practice. 'There but for the Grace of God' may apply to many of the cases Professor Grayson has drawn together from all over the world and there are many objective lessons to be learnt.

I commend Professor Grayson on his timely publication and recommend it to doctors and members of the professions allied to medicine. I also believe it worthy of serious consideration by the administrators of sport at the highest level as it highlights the importance of informed ethical standards in the regulations of sport. *Ethics, Injuries and the Law in Sports Medicine* has features that are timeless and I believe this text will become a key reference for medicine, the law and sports administration in this developing aspect of sport.

Donald A.D. Macleod.

17 March, 1999

# Preface

Brazil's international footballer Ronaldo's reported seizure suffered before the 1998 World Cup final 'has excited as much comment among doctors as among sports enthusiasts'. Thus wrote the London *Times* newspaper's medical columnist Dr Thomas Stuttatford during the week after the event on 16 July (p. 18). He explained:

> There has been discussion on which of the various relevant factors could have triggered this episode. Was it stress, the withdrawal of painkillers, prescribed for his knee or ankle, or heavy sedation?

A few days later, the *Guardian* newspaper's Rio de Janeiro correspondent, Alex Bellos, and the BBC World Service reported how:

> The team doctor Lidio Toledo has been told that he must appear before Rio's medical council to explain an alleged breach of confidentiality in suggesting to journalists that Ronaldo had suffered an epileptic fit.

Initially conceived as *Sports Medicine: Ethics and the Law* this book has become *Ethics, Injuries and the Law in Sports Medicine* to include for the first time ever a *practical* base for all Sports Medicine practitioners, through the World Medical Association (WMA) ethical guidelines for doctors involved in sport. They were formulated initially in 1981, and subsequently amended in 1987 and 1993 from a worldwide membership of approximately seventy different countries. It is an original and *practical* medico-legal book aimed to fill a gap for practitioners at all levels concerned with what is now recognized as the rapidly developing growth area of '*Sport Medicine*'. It also is a logical corollary to my earlier single chapter of *Sports Medicine and the Law* contained in Butterworths' *Sport and the Law* published in 1988 and 1994.

It does not seek to rival or compete with annually expanding shelves of sports injuries clinical or medico-legal literature. Rather, it intends to supplement them, at a time when the Academy of Medical Royal Colleges in the United Kingdom agreed in 1998 to launch a new Intercollegiate Academic Board to develop sport and exercise medicine in the United Kingdom. The Board was created to maintain and develop high standards in this area of medical care for the benefits of patients and the public, by setting and appraising standards, promoting education and training and encouraging research, as well as providing a service to those participating in sport and exercise. Initially it intended to focus 'on improving the care provided by the "touch line" doctor'.

Furthermore Medical Ethics have occupied commentators and philosophers and practitioners even before the days of Hippocrates and his immortal Oath; and twenty years ago now in 1979 Sir Roger Bannister, from his standpoint as the first four-minute mile record holder and a practising neurologist before becoming Master of Pembroke College, Oxford, wrote in his foreword to Professor Peter McIntosh's book *Fair Play: Ethics in Sport and Education*:

> It is an increasingly popular notion among many young people that we can throw off ethical and moral principles in more and more spheres of life . . . The fact of the matter is that we are faced with moral choices many times a day and if we do not notice them it must be that our intelligence or sensitivity is becoming blunted. Sport, which occupies the professional time of a few and the spare time of many, is a fit study for ethics.

This is not that book: but the World Medical Association which was created after the scientific and medical atrocities during the Second World War produced at their World Medical Assemblies successively at Lisbon, Portugal 1981, Madrid, Spain 1987, Budapest, Hungary 1993, 'ethical guidelines for physicians in order to meet the needs of sportsmen or athletes and the special circumstances in which the medical care and health guidance is given'.

Thus, for the first time, sports medicine, with its universal language like music was provided with universally based worldwide guidelines of an ethical framework to create a working structure for understanding of the law relating to medical and paramedical practices as an essential ethical element for all associated with it. Furthermore, while television and air transport have revolutionized sport and leisure at public levels from rural and urban Victorian British pastimes, transcending all social classes to become a gigantic slice of the mega international commercial entertainment leisure industry, domestic governing sporting bodies today function within a global network of international federations, exemplified by the IOC, FIFA, IRFB, ICC, IAAF, FINA. They thereby create an international form of law regulating sport worldwide, alongside medicine and music as an international language understood universally, and of comparable recognition and practicability to the World Medical Association ethical guidelines.

Medico-legal and sports medicine publications pour out from printing presses, with the regularity of sporting competitions throughout a calendar year, covering clinical and general medical areas; but this book does not attempt to challenge or compete with them. It assumes that every reader is familiar with his, or her, professional medical or paramedical professional disciplines and the sporting codes and practices applicable to their patients' activities. It is nevertheless a natural and logical corollary to what I began coincidentally, and almost symbolically, in 1953, the year when sports medicine practitioners were founding the British Association of Sport and Medicine (BASM).

During my early days of practice at the Bar, the then traditional blend of football in winter and cricket in summer had led me to prepare for publication a general text for both team games. It was based upon my schoolboy's hero-worshipping correspondence with England's cricket playing Corinthian centre-forward at the century's turn, G. O. Smith, the Gary Lineker of earlier days. A badly treated broken leg, suffered in the Oxford University soccer trials at Iffley Road, had prevented any further player participation. Entitled *Corinthians and Cricketers*, to which C. B. Fry contributed the original Foreword, it reappeared with additions in 1996 by Hubert Doggart and Gary Lineker, and an extended title *Towards a New Sporting Era*. In the early 1950s it led directly to successful professional instructions, on behalf of the then Professional Footballers' and Trainers' Union (now the PFA, the Professional Footballers' Association), to equate professional footballers' benefit testimonials on comparable terms free from tax with professional cricketers'; raising the flag for restraints of trade in Court, and in a different dimension, advocating the joint Oxford and Cambridge University F.A. Amateur Cup winning team as Pegasus on two occasions in 1951 and 1953 before 100 000 Wembley Stadium crowds to be eligible for sporting educational charitable status, with corresponding tax advantages.

Yet at no time then however, had the current sporting problems concerning violence, drugs and moral, mental and physical fitness, demanding Parliamentary and Court intervention to safeguard spectators' and players' interests at all levels, surfaced in national, international or my own personal consciousness. Today, an almost daily report internationally of injuries and/or Government or Court intrusion with areas involved with playing fields has become essential for the welfare of sport, at every level, nationally and internationally, with its impact on the health, educational and ethical values of any civilized community.

During the periods while these pages were being prepared for publication, serious injuries were recorded in the United Kingdom national media to international performers such as Alan Shearer, Robbie Fowler, Kelly Holmes, Wales' Rugby captain Gwyn Jones. The London High Court was called upon to adjudicate for a disputed drug claim between an international shot putter, Paul Edwards, against the British Athlete Federation and International Amateur Athletic Federation. A London Court of Appeal judgement sanctioned authority for Diane Modahl to progress with a substantial damages claim against the British Athlete Federation for denial of a fair hearing during a domestic tribunal investigation for an alleged drug offence of which she was exonerated on appeal. A Berlin Court room witnessed commencement of criminal prosecution proceedings for assault occasioning actual bodily harm against two doctors and four coaches with a prospect of potential prison sentences on conviction, for giving steroids to infant swimmers competing internationally for the former East German Republic. The International Amateur Athletic Federation agonized administratively over the correct sanction period of punishment for drug-related offences because of different legal court rulings from different countries in its membership; the world famous French cycling *Tour de France* tournament was overshadowed with criminally linked drug-related allegations involving arrests of medical and other team officials; the Irish Olympic swimming gold medallist, Michelle Bruin, was awaiting an International Swimming Federation (FINA) investigation result into alleged drug offences; an international lawyers' conference at Potsdam University in Germany attempted in vain to produce a formula for harmonizing sanctions for drug-related offences in all sports; and the Italian National Olympic Committee in June 1997 initiated an international legal debate for Penal Liability in Sports Activity under the title of *Guilty of Wanting to Win*, following the death at Imola of Ayrton Senna.

In concurrent developments for more physical medico-sports related problems the Football Association in London announced the establishment of a Medical Research Project, not dissimilar from that which the Scottish Rugby Union had been advocating and pursuing since 1991. The England Rugby Football Union was required to investigate an ear-biting offence during a professional competitive match which followed a comparable precedent from the American World Heavyweight boxing arena; a former Welsh international rugby prop forward, Ricky Evans, obtained an interim compensation award of £5225 (FF50 000) against a French opponent, Olivier Merle, at the High Court in Paris after a head butt described by the presiding judge as an 'act of brutality'; a disabled

American professional golfer persuaded an American Court to activate that country's disability legislation to allow him to override the United States Professional Golfers' Association (USPGA) prohibition against alleviation of his disability to prevent his being carried around the course in a golf buggy; the Hillsborough Sheffield Wednesday Stadium disaster, which caused 95 spectator fatalities in 1985, is still subject to further British Government and judicial challenges based on different evidence from what had earlier been available to a contentious Coroner's Inquest.

During the preparation of these pages the Fédération Internationale de Médecine Sportive (FIMS) produced in September 1997 a comparable but less compact Code of Ethics in Sports Medicine; and the *Lancet* reported from The University of New South Wales, Sydney, Australia, an inaugural Symposium on the Olympian Athlete relating to what an American participant from the University of California at Los Angeles, Gerald Finerman, explained as advances in diagnostic techniques and minimally invasive arthroscopic surgery, had made the treatment of elite athletes a new discipline.

Finally, as the final proof pages were being corrected, the President of the International Olympic Committee, Juan Antonio Samaranch, raised the temper of the medico-pharmacological-ethical climate when commenting in an interview with a Spanish daily newspaper and recorded in the London *Daily Telegraph* (26 July, 1998) and the BBC World Service that 'substances that do not damage a sportsman's health should not be banned'.

The reverberations from this bombshell will be seen and heard worldwide during and after these pages are published. A week later the Head of the International Olympic Medical Commission, Prince Alexandre de Merode, was recorded in the *Independent* (18 August, 1998) to have been 'appalled' after Samaranch was reported to have said he saw no harm in athletes taking certain drugs as long as they were not a threat to health.

I don't understand,

he said

> people who want to reduce the list of banned drugs are those who want doping to continue. President Samaranch has always been against doping and he has always supported the action taken by the medical commission. I know where these ideas have come from – doctors who have forgotten their professional ethics.

Not surprisingly the World Medical Association has now entered the stage, and before these pages appear a paper written by the Danish Medical Association will have been discussed by the WMA at its meeting in Ottawa (October 1998) claiming participation by doctors in drugs is as reprehensible as deciding if prisoners are able to withstand torture. The *Daily Telegraph* recorded (21 August, 1998) that:

> Doctors believe that abuse of drugs in sport is now so widespread that participants are keenly interested in finding doctors with the best reputation for masking the drug taken

and in relation to this claim the WMA's Secretary General, Dr Delon Human, explained:

> Physicians' involvement in trying to conceal the use of drugs is totally unethical.

Indeed, it is in total breach of Guideline 4, developed and explained in Chapter 5 on pages 81–90.

Finally, to complete the fall-out from this climax to the disclosures leading to renaming the international cycling Tour de France as the 'Tour de Farce', Samaranch and de Merode jointly on the same day when the WMA entered the scene, announced the creation of a two-day international conference at Lausanne on 2–3 February, 1999 for a belated attempt to regain the initiative in the never ending battle with modern international sport's escalating drug problem. The announcement including an intention to involve national government participation was tardy recognition of a global issue transcending sport's parochial territories. It accompanied the news recorded concurrently that three members of the former East German sporting establishment had been fined up to DM27 000 (DM9000 each) for damaging the health of 17 swimmers between 1979 and 1989 by giving them steroids to improve performance. The *Financial Times* (21 August, 1998) recorded:

> The conviction of doctors Ulrich Suender and Dorit Poesier and coach Peter Mattonet – the first of its kind is likely to open the door to further trials of those involved in what is believed to have been widespread, state-sponsored doping in East Germany. The Berlin court dropped charges against two other defendants.

Before publication many more similar occurrences to those summarized above, and in the pages which follow hereafter, will have been reported. The quantum of precedents from the USA and Canada, is not surprising, with their wider geographical and population areas and a generally litigation led social culture established longer than in the United Kingdom and the application to medico-sports legal principles of the general medico-legal issues, separate and apart from one special feature. This is the development in the UK of sports medicine at all medical and paramedical levels, from dedicated enthusiasts, whose professional concerns and experiences and insight *to date* have avoided any apparent public pattern of complaint about their professional sports medicine services, comparable to the USA and Canada; and the creation of the Academic Board will ensure that their standards will be maintained for less experienced and dedicated entrants to this new discipline in the future.

By its unique framework this book stands apart to bring together the differing disciplines of Ethics, Injuries, Sport, Medicine and the Law, built into it collectively together for the first time ever throughout the world. It also points the way to saving sport from its own self-destruction while the commercially corrupt competitive pressures driven by sponsored greed for prizes, prestige and profit at the domestic and international entertainment levels devastate their physiological and moral impact upon the health and attitudes of the overwhelming majority of grass roots participants seeking enjoyment, fun and pleasure from healthy recreational exercise. The Ronaldo experience may yet turn out to be a classic example of this development.

In order to introduce readers unfamiliar with, and even those who may be familiar with some, if not all of the disparate elements creating its unique interactive subject matter, I have structured the pattern of the book designedly with a progressively unfolding development in mind.

First, as a prelude to the WMA Guidelines which are the theme for the whole text I have implemented as the basis for the Introduction *Why, Now – and How?* the favourite quotation by one of Britain's most eminent and celebrated twentieth century judges and jurists, Lord Denning, from Scotland's most renowned barrister and chronicler, Sir Walter Scott:

A lawyer without history or literature is a mere working mechanic: if he possesses some knowledge of these he may venture to call himself an architect.

Thereafter Chapter 1, 'Sport and the law in the world of medicine', explains the special interaction between the disciplines in a more concentrated requirement than exists in a wider medico-legal context.

Chapters 2–10 inclusive identify and illustrate the application to sports medicine of the individual WMA Guidelines.

Chapter 11 cites and argues for a potential additional Guideline formulated by Professor Donald Mcleod, current President of the British Association for Sport and Medicine and consistent with two historic landmark articles in the *British Medical Journal* for

December 1978, which built on earlier pioneering work in the preceding twenty years from the USA and Dr John Silver at Britain's National Spinal Injuries Centre at Stoke Mandeville in Buckinghamshire. The renowned Welsh Rugby International and orthopaedic surgeon, J. P. R. Williams, identified injurious consequences of unlawful scrum collapses; one of the Welsh Rugby Union's medical advisers, Professor John Davies and his colleague Terry Gibson, explained foul play sources of injuries in their Guy's Hospital Athletics Injury Clinic; and in the final stages of preparing these pages, Canada's chair of the Canadian Centre for Ethics in Sport, Professor Andrew Pipe, published in America's *The Physician and Sports Medicine* (Professor Andrew Pipe MD) his plea for *Reviving Ethics in Sports: Time for Physicians to Act* (Appendix III).

Chapter 12 concludes with an appraisal of how all medical guidelines and legal opinions are valueless in practice to be beneficial for patients and clients without an awareness of the crucial necessity to ascertain the essential factual foundations for a correct clinical diagnosis and provable forensic evidence.

With this textual Guideline for what follows hereafter the reader should be able to thread a pathway through a new contention for what is the most important aspect of the Law relating to Sport while it hurtles towards the millennium at the public entertainment showbiz level. This is the Preamble to Dr Joseph Farber's Working Paper entitled *A code of ethics for sports medicine*. It was presented for consideration to the World Medical Association's Council's Committee on Medical Ethics in October 1980 (Appendix I) and began, with my own emphasis:

> It would be helpful to start by pointing out the *distinction between sport as a recreation*, and *competitive sport as practised by professionals*, for the doctor specialising in sport has a fundamentally different role according to which of these his patient engages in.

For 'doctor', of course, read all associated directly and indirectly with sports medicine and indeed, sport generally.

Yet this often ignored, misunderstood or frequently deliberately overlooked distinction is fundamental to comprehending the true nature of what sport may be perceived or understood to be in the dying days of the twentieth century which has stood sport on its head.

America's renowned *Sports Illustrated* 40th anniversary 1954–1994 celebration issue claimed:

> Sometime in the second half of this century, sport became the axis on which the world turns. ... There have been comparable times in history when sports have been at the centre of a culture and seemed to

dominate the landscape, whether in Greek society or what used to be the Golden Age of Sports. But ... *everything* is magnified by television.

Television and air transport have telescoped the globe; and international sporting governing body federations regulate whatever may be conceived as sport while millions worldwide who participate within it rarely pause to consider its true nature and meaning. Dr Farber did. So, too, did Sir Denis Follows CBE, former Chairman of the British Olympic Association, Secretary of the Football Association, and Treasurer of Britain's Central Council of Physical Recreation. In a potentially posthumous farewell lecture during 1983 entitled *Whither Sport* he explained:

> Sport at top level has become much more part of the entertainment world and particularly so during the past thirty years. We have reached the age where sport at top level has become almost completely show biz – the cult of the individual, high salaries, the desire to present the game as a spectacle – with more money, less sportsmanship, more emphasis on winning – and all this has largely come about through television.

He also concluded:

> After years of trying, that sport defies definition. The Sports Council tried it and gave it up as a bad job.

Three years later a United Kingdom House of Commons Environmental Committee Report in February 1986 on the workings of the Sports Council included a written memorandum from its then Director-General, John Wheatley, dated 30 October, 1985, entitled 'Financing of Sport in the United Kingdom'. It stated under the head of definition in paragraph 2:

> A study of the financing of sport produced a problem of definition. There is no single list of activities which would meet with universal agreement. Many years ago sport was felt by some to encompass hunting, shooting and fishing. A much wider view is now taken by many people,

and the same paragraph concluded with financial references 'from a variety of sources which have different definitions'.

Thus Britain's first-ever Minister with Special Responsibility for Sport, who created its role during 1962 in Mr MacMillan's Government before he became three times Lord High Chancellor as Lord Hailsham of St Marylebone, explained in his memoirs *A Sparrow's Flight*:

> In a sense there is no such thing as sport. There is only a heterogeneous list of pastimes, with different governing bodies, different

ethics and different and constantly varying needs. There are funds to pay for the training and fares of Olympic athletes, there are demands for sports centres, problems of law and order connected with sporting contests, questions relating to the safety of sports grounds, varying views about bloodsports, boxing, horse racing and many other topics.

Indeed, this breath of realism from one of the rare creative thinkers about this crucial cultural slice of modern life ties in with the 113 different non-profit making sports activities identified in Table 1.1 on page 20 which qualify for exemption for Value Added Tax purposes. It also reflects what another profound jurist, Lord Bryce, in his *Studies in History and Jurisprudence*, Vol. II, p. 181, observed:

> ... there are some conceptions which it is safer to describe than to attempt to define.

No better description can be found than what the award-winning *Daily Mail* sportswriter Ian Wooldridge explained on the never-to-be-forgotten Cliff Morgan BBC *Sport on Four* Saturday mornings radio programme following elimination of all the United Kingdom national soccer teams from the 1994 World Cup Soccer competition. He said:

> Does Sport still exist? Well it does: but you have to go out into the suburbs and shires to find it. Village cricket, soccer on Hackney Marshes, Old Boys' rugger teams getting legless afterwards, point-to-pointing, county golf, darts leagues in Dorset.

Thus, Dr Joseph Farber's distinction for creating the World Medical Association Ethical Guidelines

> ... between sport as a recreation, and competitive sport as practised by professionals,

is based on reality.

Finally, for the sports medical and paramedical practitioner a key perspective to what follows hereafter has been crystallized in the timely second edition, during 1998, while these pages were in preparation, from the litigation source of so much guidance in the particular playing field in the USA in *Sports and the Law: Text, Cases, Problems* from Professor Paul C. Weiler at Harvard Law School and Professor Gary R. Roberts at Tulane Law School. In their penultimate chapter 'Back to Torts' at page 982 they write, from their American perspective of course:

> Why are so many medical malpractice suits brought by athletes against team doctors? Is this merely symptomatic of a broader exploitation in malpractice claims? Or do special features of sports aggravate this problem? If the latter, are there any available cures?

and then they continue:

> Besides the team physician, an attractive third-party target for a tort suit by an injured player is the manufacturer of a product used in the game. . . . No sports product has been affected more by such suits than the helmets used in football, hockey and elsewhere.

with the American experience in their context. A further develop-ment of this legal penalty area (not mentioned in their text) can be seen at the end of Chapter 5 (WMA Guideline 4) where the Supreme Court of Oregon held drug manufacturers liable in negligence to a physician whose patient (albeit a non-sporting participant) was blinded by their substance (page 89): *Oksenholt v Lederle Laboratories.*

Also, and understandably not mentioned in their text dealing with the broadest basis for *Sports and the Law* transcending Sports and Medicine, Weiler and Roberts omit, in company with so many other writers in all of these areas, the World Medical Association ethical guidelines for physicians treating sportsmen or athletes which form the basis of this book. Nevertheless, their identification from their side of the Atlantic of a potential 'broader exploitation in malpractice claims' and/or 'an attractive third-party target . . . is the manufacturer of a product used in the game' points to a need for a particular recognition and awareness for and throughout these pages.

This is the existence of different juridical and jurisdictional international attitudes among the approximately seventy different member countries of the World Medical Association, and their sports related organizations and federations whose medical teams and practitioners are subject to the WMA Guidelines. For inevi-tably and concurrently, they can create different legal criteria and variations in medical practice in different parts of the world relating to the practice of sports medicine.

Accordingly, writing from The Temple in London's legal heart-land, I have tried to keep in mind throughout these pages the global perspective which must dominate the different regulatory controls from different legislative and judicial decisions of not only sports medicine, but also the wider umbrella under which it exists of medical practice generally. Thus, the monumental 924 pages of *Principles of Medical Law*, edited by Ian Kennedy and Andrew Grubb, explained in a Preface dated 1 June, 1998:

> The law in the main text is stated at 31 December 1997, although some later developments have been incorporated where possible.

A month later, on 1 July, 1998, Andrew Grubb wrote in the Preface to its *First Supplement*:

Medical law is such a fast moving subject that it has been necessary to prepare a short supplement to accompany the publication of the main text of *Principles of Medical Law*. The supplement seeks to bring the text up to date as at 1 July 1998.

A comparable urgency, at the time of writing in later 1998, does not exist for the five-dimensional *Ethics, Injuries and the Law in Sports Medicine* within the framework of the WMA Guidelines. They have stood the test of time since their inception and throughout their amendments in 1987 and 1993. Furthermore, this is confirmed by a curiously challengeable and almost ambiguous claim in the Medico-legal Issues chapter in the *Current Review of Sports Medicine*, 2nd edition, also published in 1998 in the USA with its 51 States.

From South Texas College of Law, Houston, Texas, Professor Mathew J. Mitten, JD, explained:

> Although several lawsuits have been brought against sports medicine physicians alleging malpractice, little legal precedent has been established, because most cases settle before the merits of asserted claims are judicially resolved.

The challenge to the claim and its ambiguity comes from the numerous lawsuits within and without the USA contained in these pages, and also the 1998 USA *Current Review of Sports Medicine* itself. They are all merely the tip of an unfathomable international legal iceberg which contains *evidenciary variations of a legal base*, consistent with wider *principles* of *medical law*. In other words, much legal precedent does exist for guidance to all who are concerned with the application of *differing sports medicine factual situations* to identifiable legal principles applicable throughout the world. The legal precedent can be an illustration of a comparable *factual* circumstance. It can also identify an accepted and acceptable hard core *legal principle* applicable to identifiable *evidenciary* and *factual conditions*; and here Professor Mitten is on firmer ground.

He describes the legal and evidenciary criteria applicable to sports medicine common to both sides of the Atlantic and throughout the British Commonwealth of Nations, subject to one substantive difference to be explained immediately hereafter.

From a USA perspective, he writes:

> While providing medical care to an athlete, a physician has a legal obligation to have and use the knowledge and skill ordinarily possessed and used by members of his or her speciality in good standing (depending on the state of medical science at the time such care is rendered). The law allows the medical profession to collectively determine the parameters of appropriate sports medicine care and to establish proper medical practices and treatment that should be

followed within those boundaries. In other words, a physician must adhere to customary or accepted sports medicine practices within his or her speciality. The medical standard of care, which must be established by physician expert testimony, is the legal standard of care in a malpractice case.

Anglo-Saxon practitioners of the Common Law throughout the world will recognize in that citation the formula laid down more than forty years ago by Mr Justice McNair in *Bolam v Friern Hospital Management Committee* [1957] 2 All ER 118, and recently refined and reaffirmed by the House of Lords in *Bolitho v City and Hackney Health Authority* [1997] 4 All ER 771. Lord Brown-Wilkinson explained in more detail than is necessary here for the general explanatory global WMA Guidelines purpose:

> In the *Bolam* case itself, McNair J stated that the defendant had to have acted in accordance with the practice accepted as proper by a 'responsible body of medical men'. Later he referred to a 'standard of practice recognized as proper by a competent reasonable body of opinion' ... the court has to be satisfied that the exponents of the body of opinion relied upon can demonstrate that such opinion has a logical basis.

The one substantive difference between Britain and many other medico-legal jurisdictions is expressed crisply in *Principles of Medical Law* (1998) edited by Kennedy and Grubb at page 166 in para. 3.124:

> The North American doctrine of 'informed consent' (always something of a misnomer) is not part of English law.

Four years earlier J. K. Mason and R. A. McCall Smith from over the Scottish border in the 4th edition of *Law and Medical Ethics* developed this briefly:

> Within the British Commonwealth, there are decisions ranging from the endorsement of the deliberate medical lie to the acceptance of the extreme patient-orientated approach which emphasizes complete disclosure of risk. The United States with its 51 independent jurisdictions, provides a useful overall view. Although a majority of the states still apply a professional standard, there is a recognizable drift towards that of the prudent patient.

These cultural and socio-medicolegal differences are even more important for awareness by the peripatetic sports medical and paramedical practitioner travelling around the world on the modern television orientated international sports circuit, at risk to be at service in emergency even beyond the calls of sporting duties. The essentiality of adequate insurance cover is self-evident; and while the American litigation climate has yet to hit Britain's sporting medical scene, these above citations recall the opening page of my earlier Preface to Butterworths' 2nd (1994) edition of *Sport and the Law*:

> ... sport, with medicine and music, like Tauber's song, goes round the world; and from across the Atlantic, one of America's greatest gifts to Anglo-Saxon culture, as judge, jurist, legal historian and practitioner, Oliver Wendell Holmes, Jr, explained in the opening paragraph of his tome on *The Common Law*, with a theme comparable to Glenn Miller's *Moonlight Serenade*, 'The life of the law has not been logic: it has been experience'. He echoed an earlier attribution to the English sage of the previous century, Dr Samuel Johnson; 'The Law is the last Result of Publick Wisdom, acting upon publick Experience' (from *Dr Johnson and the Law* by Sir Arnold McNair KC).

Experience for all medico-legal writers demands a final whistle for the state of play and applicable law, even in such daily developing disciplines as ethics, injuries, medicine, sport and the law. Coincidence and the Great Umpire in the Sky combined to bring down the curtain almost symbolically on the 50th anniversary of the United Nations signature of the Declaration of Human Rights, 10 December, 1948 [1998]; from the days of sporting innocence at the public entertainment level before drugs, violence, cheating, corruption and media distorting began to dominate the *public entertainment* which sadly fills the stage today, and overshadow the grass roots perception of international sport and recreation, as they appear to apply for the law as stated on 10 December, 1998.

Edward Grayson
9–12 Bell Yard
Temple Bar
London

# Acknowledgements

The preparation and compilation of these pages result directly from the earlier single chapter in *Sports Medicine and the Law* in Butterworths' two editions of *Sport and the Law* published in 1988 and 1994, and they could not have been possible without the sustained support and encouragement from all sources cited in the text, Appendices and References. In particular, I wish to acknowledge the inspiration from Dr Delon Human and Professor Donald Macleod for their Forewords, and their respective organizations, the World Medical Association, Inc., and the British Association of Sport and Medicine, and also the Sports Section of the Royal Society of Medicine. The library and staff there, and also their associated colleagues, have always responded with experience and insight at the libraries of the Honourable Societies of Middle and Inner Temple, the National Sports Medicine Institute, the Sports Council, *Times*, *Daily Telegraph*, *Yorkshire Post*, *Rugby World*, and the BBC World Service Sports Section.

I am particularly grateful for special permission to reproduce and update the tabulated lists of issues and cases from the texts of *Sport and the Law* by kind permission of the publisher, Butterworths, and also to my present publisher Butterworth-Heinemann and their book production department for careful and skilful editorial guidance and for arranging the List of Cases, References and the Index.

Finally, a special word of thanks is due to my professional colleagues and staff at Chambers, headed first by Edmund Lawson, QC, and more latterly by D. Anthony Evans, QC, under the Senior Clerkship of Gary Reed, for helping me to balance the daily and nightly demands of authorship with daily and nightly practice at the Bar from 9–12 Bell Yard, Temple Bar, London.

# Abbreviations

| | |
|---|---|
| ABA | Amateur Boxing Association |
| ACPSM | Association of Chartered Physiotherapists in Sports Medicine |
| BAF | British Athletic Federation |
| BASES | British Association of Sport and Exercise Sciences |
| BASM | British Association of Sport and Medicine |
| BBB of C | British Boxing Board of Control |
| BMA | British Medical Association |
| BOA | British Olympic Association |
| BOMC | British Olympic Medical Centre |
| BSAC | British Sub Aqua Club |
| CCPR | Central Council of Physical Recreation |
| CT | Computerized Tomography |
| FA | Football Association |
| FIFA | Federation of International Football Associations |
| FIMS | Fédération Internationale de Médecine Sportive |
| FINA | Fédération Internationale de Natation Amateur |
| GMC | General Medical Council |
| IAAF | International Amateur Athletic Federation |
| ICC | International Cricket Commission |
| IOC | International Olympic Committee |
| IRFB | International Rugby Football Board |
| MCC | Marylebone Cricket Club |
| MOSA | Medical Officers of Schools Association |
| MRI | Magnetic Resonance Imaging |
| NCA | National Cricket Association |
| PFA | Professional Footballers Association |
| PNS | Persistent Negative State |
| RYA | Royal Yachting Association |
| TCCB | Test and Country Cricket Board |
| VAT | Value Added Tax |
| WMA | World Medical Association |
| WTA | World Tennis Association |

# Introduction: Why now – and how?

## WHY NOW?

*Preamble*

In October 1980 a 'working paper' under the title *A code of ethics for sports medicine* was presented for consideration by the World Medical Association Council Session in Munich, by Dr Joseph Farber, Chairman of the Council's Committee on Medical Ethics. In its *Preamble* he hit the key note for understanding the true nature of sport *at all levels* by:

> pointing out the distinction between sport as a recreation, and competitive sport as practised by professionals, for the doctor specialising in sports medicine has a fundamentally different role according to which of these his patient engages in.
>
> For recreational sport, the doctor has first and foremost to be on the lookout for contraindications to the desired sporting activity as much before as during the event.
>
> The doctor must always be in a position to advise against participation in a sport which, whether through age or illness, has become harmful to his patient. The work of this doctor will bring him up against various obstacles, not least of which is the argument whether sporting activities really do have a beneficial effect on health.

Thereafter, in the manner to be seen in the full text at Appendix 1 to these pages Dr Farber outlined the doctor's different roles in competitive professional and international sport while emphasizing the distinction between Amateur and Competitive professional sports with an awareness which is more often overlooked than identified when sport is considered generally at any level, on any occasion. A year later, based upon that 'working paper' in 1981, The World Medical Association (WMA) drafted ethical guidelines for doctors involved in sport in 1981 (with subsequent amendments in 1987 and 1993). They are used here for the first time ever as a coherent framework within which to explain:

1

1 The ethical framework within which they are required to operate for sports medicine doctors, dentists, nurses, sports physiotherapists, podiatrists and all other sports paramedical services, including St John's and St Andrew's services coaches, participators and their administrators.

2 How, within that ethical framework, the traditional medico-legal criteria apply to this developing area, both nationally and internationally.

3 Why and how the global disciplines of sport, medicine, ethics, injuries and the law, built into the title of this book, should combine at every level of public entertainment and private participation to protect (and prevent the commercial and bureaucratic exploitation of) the health and welfare of participators in international sport and recreation: the twentieth century's greatest cultural and social explosion.

4 How the fall-out from the explosion of international sport and recreation has created two concurrent cultural gaps comparable to D'Israeli's *Two Nations* and C. P. Snow's *Two Cultures of Art and Science*:

    (a) that of the division between sport and recreation at the public, entertainment, media-orientated and commercial levels on the one hand, and the fun-seeking, healthy, recreational grassroots (but nevertheless competitive) and educational dimension on the other; and

    (b) the even more insidious gap between those with respect for the Rule of Law in Sport (reflective of the rule of law in society generally) and those demonstrating an unconcealed contempt for such doctrinal idealism, evidenced by the mounting casualties in breach of road traffic regulations and comparable breaches of the laws of sport, where in each discipline, medical evidence provides damning proof of callous social and sporting misconduct.

Because the essential clinical basis for sports medicine will always be prevention and cure, the subject is linked inevitably to sports injuries, which in turn are directly related to sporting activity. In addition, the subject must address conventional illnesses which transcend sport, but which nevertheless affect performance, such as asthma or psychological problems. Without identification of the injuries which sports medicine and its ethical and legal framework must always seek to prevent and cure, the subject – and this book – would be as arid and unrealistic as an attempted assessment of the equestrian industries without the horses.

Today, sports medicine has developed to become an identifiable area of practice in its own right, from a Cinderella section of the medical and paramedical professions, experienced as a hobby alongside a more general or specialized medical purpose, depending upon which area of recognized medical knowledge a doctor, surgeon, physician, physiotherapist, podiatrist or any other practitioner offers his or her services, to its present elevated level in early 1998, in the United Kingdom. The Academy of Medical Royal Colleges created an Intercollegiate Board of Sport and Exercise Medicine, *inter alia* to 'encourage best practice in the diagnosis and management of sports and exercise related clinical problems'.

Contrary to general belief and understanding within as well as without the legal profession in the UK, which created the modern sporting explosion, the law has been invoked for more than a century in the Courts to protect injured victims of misconduct – off as well as on the fields, and for even longer periods in Parliament – for defence of the realm and in the interests of public health. Thus, a collapsed grandstand at the historic Cheltenham Race Week Festival in 1866, causing injuries (but happily no fatalities) among the spectators, and a football field fatality during play at Ashby-de-la-Zouch in 1878, led to appropriate legal redress (see, respectively, *Francis v Cockerell* [1870] LR 5 QB 501 and *R v Bradshaw* (1878) 14 Cox CC 83). More than 650 years earlier, Parliament seemed almost to have anticipated the modern position when football was forbidden: first, in 1314, as leading to a breach of the peace and again in 1349, because it discouraged archery practice – which naturally enough led to fears for the effective defence of the realm.

In the aftermath of the First World War, following 1918, an inevitable acceleration in the medical alleviation of military suffering led to an awareness of the need to share and exchange experiences and knowledge among sports medical practitioners. This resulted in the formation of what is now known as the Fédération Internationale de Médecine Sportive (FIMS) in 1928. The Second World War, with its disabled legatees returning to a more widely recognized sports-orientated society, provided the incentive for the development of national and international disabled sports organizations, to co-exist concurrently with the development of sports medicine for able-bodied participants.

A further development in the years following the Second World War, with its medical outrages and breaches of conventional medical ethics, was the foundation of the WMA in 1947. The WMA's overriding objective was the harmonizing of international attitudes to doctors, which began with a modernized version of the Hippocratic oath and an International Code of Medical Ethics (the Declaration of Geneva – see pages 16–18 *infra*). Subsequent declarations have gained international acceptance for various ethical medical problems which have emerged in the sporting area; for example, the Declaration of Helsinki, which concerned doctors intending to embark upon any experimental scheme of treatment.

In the UK, the British Association for Sports Medicine (BASM) was formed in 1953. It was followed in 1961 by the British Sports Association for the Disabled. Twenty years later, the first WMA ethical guidelines (initially 1–12) were established. At the 45th World Medical Assembly at Budapest, in October 1993, they were prefaced by an introduction:

> The WMA has drafted and recommends the following [1–13] ethical guidelines for physicians in order to meet the needs of the sportsmen or athletes and the special circumstances in which the medical care and health guidance is given.

It consequently established the thirteen guidelines, given below:

1   The physician who cares for sportsmen or athletes has an ethical responsibility to recognize the special physical and mental demands placed upon them by their performance in sports activities.

2   When the sports participant is a child or an adolescent, the physician must give first consideration to the participant's growth and stage of development.

   2.1   The physician must ensure that the child's stage of growth and development, as well as his or her general condition of health can absorb the rigours of the training and competition without jeopardizing the normal physical or mental development of the child or adolescent.

   2.2   The physician must oppose any sports or athletic activity that is not appropriate to the child's stage of growth and development or general condition of health. The physician must act in the best interest of the health of the child or adolescent, without regard to any other interest or pressure from any other source.

3   When the sports participant is a professional sportsman or athlete and derives livelihood from that activity, the physician should pay due regard to the occupational medical aspects involved.

4   The physician should oppose the use of any method which is not in accordance with professional ethics, or which might be harmful to the sportsman or athlete using it, especially:

   4.1   Procedures which artificially modify blood constituents or biochemistry.

   4.2   The use of drugs or other substances whatever their nature and route of administration, including central-nervous-system stimulants or depressants and procedures which artificially modify reflexes.

4.3 Induced alterations of will or general mental outlook.

4.4 Procedures to mask pain or other protective symptoms if used to enable the sportsman or athlete to take part in events when lesions or signs are present which make his participation inadvisable.

4.5 Measures which artificially change features appropriate to age and sex.

4.6 Training and taking part in events when to do so would not be compatible with preservation of the individual's fitness, health or safety.

4.7 Measures aimed at an unnatural increase or maintenance of performance during competition. Doping to improve an athlete's performance is unethical.

5 The physician should inform the sportsman or athlete, those responsible for him, and other interested parties, of the conscquences of the procedures he is opposing, guard against their use, enlist the support of other physicians and other organizations with the same aim, protect the sportsman or athlete against any pressures which might induce him to use these methods and help with supervision against these procedures.

6 The sports physician has the duty to give his objective opinion on the sportsmen or athletes' fitness or unfitness clearly and precisely, leaving no doubt as to his conclusions.

7 In competitive sports or professional sports events, it is the physician's duty to decide whether the sportsman or athlete can remain on the field or return to the game. This decision cannot be delegated to other professionals or to other persons. In the physician's absence these individuals must adhere strictly to the instructions he has given them, priority always being given to the best interests of the sportsman's or athlete's health and safety, and not the outcome of the competition.

8 To enable him to carry out his ethical obligations the sports physician must see his authority fully recognized and upheld, particularly wherever it concerns the health, safety and legitimate interests of the sportsman or athlete, none of which can be prejudiced to favour the interests of any third party whatsoever.

9 The sports physician should endeavour to keep the patient's personal physician fully informed of facts relevant to his treatment. If necessary he should collaborate with him to ensure that the sportsman or athlete does not exert himself in ways detrimental to his health and does not use potentially harmful techniques to improve his performance.

10 In sports medicine, as in all other branches of medicine, professional confidentiality must be observed. The right to privacy over medical attention the sportsman or athlete has received must be

protected, especially in the case of professional sportsmen or athletes.

11   The sports doctor must not be party to any contract which obliges him to reserve particular forms of therapy solely and exclusively for any one sportsman or athlete or group of sportsmen or athletes.

12   It is desirable that sports physicians from foreign countries, when accompanying a team in another country, should enjoy the right to carry out their specific functions.

13   The participation of a sports physician is desirable when sports regulations are being drawn up.

The thrust and focus of these thirteen guidelines are targeted inevitably and understandably towards the doctor–patient relationship, with an inevitable potential applicability to other sports health professionals. Breach may provide evidence of negligence in a way analogous to breaches of the Highway Code in road traffic cases. Complaints arising from serious breaches may attract the attention of the British or any other national equivalent to its GMC. Nevertheless, the unique purpose behind them involves, additionally, an overriding and inherent relationship with sport itself, which demands a framework to transcend and bind all others to preserve its integrity as a basis for healthy recreation, education and fun in a rapidly developing commercially orientated sport-related competitive society. This ideal was crystallized in 1990 by the President of the BASM, Honorary Medical Advisor to the Scottish Rugby Union and Professor of Sports Medicine at Aberdeen University since January 1998, Donald Macleod (Macleod, 1990) as a proposed Guideline 14 in *The Doctor's Contribution to Safety in Sport* (*Medicine, Sport and the Law*), Blackwell Scientific Publications, p. 61 at 65–6:

14.1 Doctors involved in sport have an ethical and legal duty to provide competent professional services and to ensure that they practice medicine to a high standard with appropriate facilities.

14.2 The doctor has an additional ethical responsibility with regard to the prevention of injury by advising that appropriate equipment is worn by players, the environment is safe, and vulnerable individuals do not participate in an event when there is a risk of aggravating a primary injury or sustaining a second, invariably more serious, injury.

14.3 If a doctor recognizes a pattern of events leading to injury, he has an ethical duty to draw this to the attention of the players, coaches and legislators, in the hope that this pattern can be broken and the injuries minimized.

14.4 On occasion, the doctor may be faced with a situation where an injury has resulted from violence outside the rules of the game.

This may occur as a result of careless or thoughtless play, but may be the result of deliberate cheating, recklessness or violence and, in these circumstances, the doctor has a duty both to treat the injured player and to protect other players from similar violence by informed liaison with the relevant official in the event club or sport and the individuals concerned (NB while preserving professional confidentiality through anonymity).

The last two criteria were consistent with the evidence provided in the *British Medical Journal* on 23–30 December, 1978 from two land mark contributions by John Davies and Terry Gibson, who recorded how 'foul play might have caused as many as [31 per cent] of all reported [rugby] injuries' in their Guy's Hospital Athletics Injuries Clinic. Similarly, J. P. R. Williams, in his capacity both as one of Wales' international full-backs and a surgical registrar with Professor B. McKibbin at the Department of Traumatic and Orthopaedic Surgery at Cardiff Royal Infirmary, warned of the physical dangers from deliberate scrum collapses.

By 1990, after the second (1981) but before the third (1993) version of the WMA guidelines, two significant general developments were recorded. A book entitled *Medical Negligence* was published under the editorship of Michael Powers, a barrister and doctor, and Nigel H. Harris, a consultant orthopaedic surgeon (1990). The book comprised a collection of nearly forty chapters by highly qualified specialists drawn from both the medical and legal professions. As the editors explained in the preface to the first edition written as at November 1989:

The decline in the teaching of legal medicine has been deplored by Professor A. Keith Mant (1986, *British Medical Journal* 29 Nov.). Both the educational committee of the General Medical Council and the advisory committee on the medical training of the Commission of the European Community have stated that newly qualified doctors should have an adequate knowledge of the laws concerning medical practice and more time should be spent in the undergraduate medical curriculum on ethical and legal aspects of medical practice.

Towards the end of the same year, 1990, a working party of the Medical Ethics Committee of the British Medical Association, which had been influential in establishing the WMA, was created with what it described ultimately as:

... the ambitious task of conducting a review of the Association's published ethical advice and producing 'practical advice with extrapolation of the philosophical principles in order to guide doctors in any aspects of their practice where ethical considerations arise'.

Three years later, in 1993, the committee published *Medical Ethics Today: Its Practice and Philosophy* (BMA Medical Ethics Committee working party, 1993).

The Introduction explained:

This book is intended to be a practical guide which reflects contemporary ethical thinking. It is written primarily for doctors but we hope that other people will find it useful. Its approach is patient-centred. Emphasis is given to promoting a balanced partnership between doctors and patients, which means that effective communication (which includes listening to the patient as well as giving him or her information) must be seen as a key component of practical medical ethics. Increasingly, doctors play a role within a team of professionals and so attention is also given to inter-professional dialogue.

The fundamental principles observed by the medical profession remain constant but their application to newly evolving situations requires debate. ... In many cases, doctors' enquiries are more mundane than the ethical issues which philosophers, lawyers and bio-ethicists debate. Since doctors tend to need a quick and workable solution for an immediate case, we focus on a practical response to these common questions but this process inevitably brings in reference to philosophy and law. ... Even superficially simple queries, such as how much information to give a patient, or whether children can choose treatment for themselves [A. Franck and H. Olagnier (1996) see later p. 68] cannot be answered fully without mentioning how legal cases and bio-ethical discussions are influencing medical practice and vice versa.

Furthermore, the prosaic questions cannot be completely separated from the major ethical dilemmas. The way in which those questions are answered, and the dilemmas resolved, must be informed by the same strands of reasoning. The responses to both the day-to-day questions, and the major ethical ones, usually reflects among other things, a judgement about the fundamental nature of the doctor–patient relationship.

That relationship is as much at the heart of sports medicine as it is for all general medical and paramedical standards. Nevertheless, a moment's thought will identify how, alongside the different specialists within medical and paramedical practice generally, different sports participants (with their different recreational and competitive age groups, disabilities, sex, and different sports and team groups) demand different levels of experience and expertise. For in addition to accidents in the home, from road traffic, and other transport injuries on air, land, and sea, no human activity produces so many injuries demanding specialist medical and paramedical attention as the world of sport and its associated areas of physical education and recreation. No comprehensive database for sports-related injury statistics will ever be available, if only because analogously to road traffic and other criminal offences, not all are ever reported or recorded. In the early 1990s, however, a British Sports Council's Sheffield University commissioned survey concluded in its 'Summary of the injuries and exercise main report – national study of the epidemiology of exercise related injury illness':

> Six million new sports injuries require treatment each year. Accident and Emergency departments are well equipped to deal with the more serious injuries, but family doctors may be less familiar with the management of sports injuries. To help reduce costs and improve effectiveness, the way in which sports injuries are managed should be reviewed. NHS Sports Injury Clinics may be needed to fill the gaps.

Six years later, a leading article in the *British Journal of Sports Medicine* from Robin Knill-Jones (June 1997 at pp. 95–6) recorded that:

> Sports related injuries form a significant part of the workload of the National Health Service. Patients with acute injuries account for between 3.9% and 7.1% of total attendances at casualty departments, and a higher proportion of attendances – 28% by children. An unknown proportion of these injuries go on to become chronic or recurrent problems which later involve orthopaedic clinics or general practitioners. Clearly, there is an unmet need for expert advice and treatment, for which, for whatever reason, NHS resources are unavailable.

Thus, it may be argued that sports medicine (and its ethical criteria), with its uniquely complex and rarely recognized general and specialist multi-disciplinary requirements, which are rarely understood within both sport and society and medicine generally, stands apart from other medical and paramedical areas. This also reflects the clear division between sport as a branch of the entertainment industry and sport in its health and education role, with or without a competitive framework. Indeed, perhaps this is why, three years earlier, the BMA's publication *Medical Ethics Today* (BMA Medical Ethics Committee working party, 1993) had ignored them. That publication in turn had explained analogously, but without specifying sport, the inevitable ethical and legal conflicts experienced by team doctors, while nevertheless identifying in detail in its section 9 under the title 'Doctors with Dual Obligations' a tranche concerned specifically with occupational health; community physicians; police surgeons; prison doctors;

doctors in the armed forces; doctors as company directors; media doctors, and those concerned with medical examinations for insurance and employment. Further, it was claimed in the Preface to *ABC of Sports Medicine* (May, 1995) that: 'Our aim is to increase the general understanding of doctors who have an interest in sports medicine but who do not consider themselves specialists.' However, that publication also omitted any references to the WMA guidelines, medico-legal criteria or ethics. It concluded:

> There are now many courses available in sports medicine and exercise science, and the recent initiative of the medical colleges of the United Kingdom of establishing an intercollegiate faculty of sports medicine does imply that training in sports medicine is being taken seriously.

Yet that training – and, indeed, that 'general understanding of doctors who have an interest in sports medicine but who do not consider themselves specialists' and even those who do consider themselves to be specialists – is incomplete without an awareness or recognition of the WMA guidelines and of how they may interact, with 'reference to philosophy and law', as explained in *Medical Ethics Today* (BMA Medical Ethics Committee working party, 1993). A year later, however, in 1994, a BMA annual representative meeting 'deplored that the BMA does not have a policy (i) for the promotion of sports medicine [and] (ii) for the representation of doctors involved in the sports medical field', and in 1996 the BMA published *Sport and exercise medicine: policy and provision* (BMA Board of Science and Education, 1996), and included the WMA ethical guidelines in an appendix, albeit without significant comment.

## HOW IT HAPPENED

Any attempt to mark out areas of unchartered territory begins definitively. In the global village which now encompasses international sport at both public and private levels, demarcation lines for sports medicine vary in different parts of the world. The then President of the FIMS, W. Hollman explained for an opening section in the *Olympic Book of Sports Medicine* (1988) at p. xi entitled 'The Definition and Scope of Sports Medicine':

> The term 'sports medicine' is a traditional name which no longer corresponds to the special field of sports medicine as we see it today. The first modern definition was made in 1958 on the occasion of the foundation of the Institute for Cardiology and Sports Medicine,

Cologne: Sports medicine includes those theoretical and practical branches of medicine which investigate the influence of exercise, training and sport on healthy and ill people, as well as the effects of lack of exercise, to produce useful results for prevention, therapy, rehabilitation, and the athlete.' This definition was adopted by the FIMS Scientific Commission in 1977.

Accordingly, prevention stands firmly in the foreground of today's sports medicine.

More recently, however, this definition was considered incomplete by the Scottish Royal Colleges' Board for Sports Medicine: they expanded it with the following criteria and a commentary on the key differences (Scottish Royal Colleges' Board for Sports Medicine, 1989):

Sports Medicine is a discipline which includes the study of theoretical and practical branches of the relevant basic sciences and medicine which investigate, document and measure the influence of life-style, exercise, training and sport – or their lack – on both healthy and physically or psychologically ill or handicapped people in order to produce useful results for the prevention of disease or injury, treatment, rehabilitation and improvement in education, health and overall performance of the individual and society.

The key differences arising from the 1977 definition are that:

1   it includes basic sciences;

2   it investigates, documents and measures;

3   it widens 'ill' to include physically ill, psychologically ill, and handicapped;

4   it includes education;

5   it deals generally with society.

Six years after the FIMS Scientific Commission's adoption of the 1958 Cologne definition in 1977, a more simplistic definition was formulated by two Swedish sports medical practitioners and teachers, Dr Lars Peterson and Dr Per Renström, in *Sports Injuries: Their Prevention and Treatment* (1983), without measuring results or commenting on the prevalence of sedentary lifestyles in modern society:

Sports medicine encompasses the following elements: preparation and training, prevention of injuries and illness, diagnosis and treatment of injuries and illness, and rehabilitation and return to active participation in sport. This definition relates to the athlete, the sport, sporting equipment and diagnostic instrumentation.

Furthermore, under the heading of characteristics of sports, they targeted the direction which every sports medical practitioner at every level should take:

> Different sports make different demands on the athlete. Competitive sport perhaps involves an increased risk of injury, but some people have a positive need to participate at this level and gain great satisfaction from doing so. Top athletes are often held up as examples to the young who are encouraged to attend sports grounds and running tracks as a result. Also top level sport arouses great public interest and plays an important part in the everyday life of many people, so is not to be discouraged.
>
> Regardless of the level at which it is played, each sport is unique in terms of the demands it places on participants and its special characteristics which can cause both overuse and traumatic injuries.

A vivid illustration of the scope and range for potential differentials in the medical requirements of different sporting disciplines can be seen from the list of 113 differing sporting activities in the UK whose non-profit-making sections qualify for Value Added Tax (VAT) exemption under the UK Treasury Notice (see Table 1.1 on p. 20) published in 1994. A more detailed categorization of this list, for clinical purposes is given below (pp. 59–60: in Chapter 2 when considering the WMA Guidelines:

> The physician who cares for sportsmen or athletes has an ethical responsibility to recognize the special physical and mental demands placed upon them by their performance in sports activities.

Finally, two further practical sources (one from an American–Welsh combination and the other from Oxford's citadel) place the WMA guidelines within the framework of a developing dimension, leading Donald Macleod, the current President of the BASM (Macleod, 1996) to advocate that:

> ... sports medicine should be brought under the umbrella of a recognised body with an accredited higher training programme . . .
> The time has come to establish a faculty or association of sport and exercise medicine for medical graduates with an appropriate group of royal colleges and their faculties acting as patron.

In 1996 the Academy of Medical Royal Colleges joined a small working group to consider how further to progress the developments in the half century since the foundation of the WMA in 1947, and in 1989, three practitioners – Arnold Williams, FRCR FRCS, Consultant Radiologist, Cardiff Royal Infirmary; Roger Evans, FRCP, Consultant in Accident & Emergency Medicine, Cardiff Royal Infirmary; and Paul D. Shirley, MD PA, Consultant

Orthopaedic Surgeon, Jacksonville, Florida in the valuable Preface to their *Imaging of Sports Injuries* (1989) stated that:

> The past three or four decades have seen immense changes in sports and allied leisure activities. The number of sports open to general participation has multiplied and along with this have gone major developments in the provision of sporting facilities. An increase in prosperity and a greater amount of leisure time together with an urge to maintain fitness has resulted in many more people continuing or restarting athletic activities beyond their days in full-time education.
>
> Thirty years ago the number of participants involved in tae-kwando or karate in the Western world would have been negligible, but today many thousands of people are active in these and other martial arts. Some events such as the triathlon were unheard of in the 1950s, as were activities such as windsurfing or skateboarding, which are common today. Sports such as squash have seen a major increase in the number of participants and there has been a positive explosion in the size of the fields for marathons and half-marathons.

Those more recently recognized activities create a different dimension and development from what might have been anticipated in the aftermath of the Second World War. Williams, Evans and Shirley continued:

> There have always been 'high risk' sports such as mountaineering and skiing but in recent years many others have appeared and become popular including parachuting, hang-gliding and cross-country racing on a variety of all-terrain vehicles. This has resulted in an increase in the number of serious sports-related injuries, particularly to regions such as the head, neck and spine.
>
> Whilst there has been this surge in the number of 'amateur' sportsmen and women, the world of the 'professional' athlete, paid or unpaid, has undergone equally radical changes. In the 1980s competition is fiercer and the financial rewards are far greater than ever before; consequently the degree of dedication required to reach the very top is now all-consuming. The day of the Corinthian has passed and the time when those selected for an international team turned up with their kit on a Saturday morning to play in the afternoon has long gone. Sport at the top is now a year round, full-time occupation.

This typically superficial reference to 'the day of the Corinthian has passed' reflects a possible general unawareness throughout the world that a celebrated amateur English soccer club which still competes in Southern England, Corinthian-Casuals, has given its name to the English language as 'The Corinthian ideal', to be a benchmark for true values in sport, recently confirmed by its citation in the 1997 obituaries and memorial tributes to the great soccer and rugby heroes, Denis Compton and Wilf Wooller. Rachel Heyhoe-Flint, hockey international and former England ladies cricket captain, in an interview early in 1998 on Cliff Morgan's BBC Radio Four's *Sport on Four*, identified the Corinthian concept within sport as 'self-fulfilment for fun, companionship and healthy recreational exercise'. A few weeks later Britain's *genuine* sports loving former Prime Minister John Major referred to it three times in a similar vein, and a further example may be found in Peter Goss, the round-the-world yachtsman, who sacrificed the chance of a prize by diverting his competition course to save the life of a fellow yachtsman in distress consistent with the Rule of Law for the Sea.

Various associations of sports medicine in many countries do foster interest amongst their fellow practitioners in sports-related problems, and this has often been against a tide of feeling that regards such damage as self-inflicted, an injury that can be best 'cured' by the patient giving up his or her sport. Thus, Williams, Evans and Shirley in their Preface further explain:

> Most doctors who are not involved in the treatment of athletes have little idea of how much time and effort top-line performers put into their training; 20 to 30 hours a week in the pool or 120 miles of road work is not uncommon, and this may be in association with an attempt to hold down a job or to keep up with a full-time academic course.

A comparable position exists for those concerned with all aspects of the performing arts; ballet, music, singing, thespians, as amateurs or professionals. They all require specialist medical services for effective treatment and preventive medicine as great as the active sports participant in a global village shrunk by television and transport facilities. Their demands were undreamed of when the pioneers, from Simpson with chloroform, Madame Curie with radiology, Pasteur and immunology down to our own century and Banting, Best and Macleod with insulin, Harold Gillies and Archibald McIndoe for plastic surgery, the triumphs of Chain, Fleur and Fleming for penicillin, and Salk and Sabin for polio, were pushing back the frontiers with their vision and creations.

Thus Williams, Evans and Shirley (1989) brought their own modern perspective into focus with a conclusion explaining the inevitable advances of applicable equipment for sports medicine. They also point out the age range of sports participants gives rise to specific issues:

> Whilst we accept that some of the injuries sustained by athletes, such as torn menisci, do occur in the general population, other injuries are specifically related to the heavy physical demands that athletic men

and women place upon their bodies. In their drive to succeed many younger athletes sustain injuries to immature skeletons which give rise to problems both immediately and in later life. The current vogue for increased activity in people aged over 40 years, in the belief that this benefits the cardiovascular system, also produces difficulties. In both the 'paediatric' and 'geriatric' athlete, injuries occur in which the diagnosis may remain obscure for long periods.

Arriving at a diagnosis in these patients has been made easier by the advances in imaging techniques that have appeared in recent years. The plain radiograph may now be supplemented by isotope bone scanning (scintigraphy), thermography, xeroradiography, computerized tomography (CT), high quality ultrasound (US), and most recently magnetic resonance imaging (MRI).

Continuing this theme, the comprehensive *Oxford Textbook of Sports Medicine* edited in 1994 by Mark Harries, Clyde Williams, William D. Skanish and Lyle J. Micheli, while omitting all references to ethical and legal issues, states in the Preface:

Sports medicine has evolved over the last 50 years from a core activity of treating injuries to one which now uses a multidisciplinary approach to the care of those injured whilst participating in sport. The rationale for this approach (and the legitimate claim on the title 'sports medicine') is that those who look after the injured are professionally obliged to offer advice on how injuries can be both treated and avoided.

Practitioners in all branches of sports medicine must now be well informed about those activities which have the potential to lead to injury. Understanding the physical and physiological demands that heavy and sustained activity places on participants in sport, whatever their age, requires a special knowledge of the adaptive responses to exercise.

In the Foreword to that volume, Sir Roger Bannister from his triple standpoint as athlete, doctor, and head of college, hoped that such a 'much needed comprehensive textbook of sports medicine' will 'also encourage examining authorities in medicine and surgery to include questions related to sports medicine in finals papers and higher examinations as a spur to raising standards of diagnosis and treatment'.

With that ultimate aim, he had earlier explained:

There are several reasons why the standard of sports medicine has lagged behind that of general medicine. First, when clinics are overcrowded, neither the consultant nor other patients may relish the notion of an athlete, injured, as they might see it, as a result of voluntary activity, being granted priority for urgent treatment. Second, since sports medicine cannot be easily defined or circumscribed, confusion arises which lowers standards of care. Sports medicine encompasses cardiology, respiratory medicine, orthopaedic surgery, traumatology and many other specialties. For years the existence of clinics for sports medicine in Britain had depended too much on the individual enthusiasm of dedicated specialists, who were prepared to create, often in their own time, clinics adjusted to suit the needs of athletes. I take the view that general medicine and surgery have a duty to learn from study of the diverse range of acute sports injury, so that the lessons can be applied to the management of traumatic injuries which also occur in other circumstances. Moreover, sport usually provides for the sports physician an enthusiastic subject, eager to regain his capacity to compete as soon as possible, which is not always true of other patients. Sports medicine specialists can also advise governing bodies of sport on the best ways to organize complex competitive rules in order to reduce the possibility of injuries. ... With some 25% of the population, including children and students, now regularly taking part in sport, the problem of treatment of injuries can no longer be regarded as a 'Cinderella' area of medicine.

If practitioners of this evolving discipline are to honour the traditions of conduct which guide the standards of any self-respecting cadre of practitioners, they need look no further than the WMA guidelines, formulated to guide the practice of medicine within sport. The late Professor A. J. Ayer, one time Wykeham Professor of Logic in the University of Oxford, was a devoted follower of Tottenham Hotspur and Middlesex County Cricket Club. In the first of his Gifford Lectures (delivered at St Andrews University in 1972–73, under the title of '*Philosophy and Science*'), he pointed out:

Ethics is indeed concerned with human conduct, but it is not descriptive of human conduct, in the way that psychology and sociology are. It can be prescriptive, but its interest is rather in what lies behind the prescriptions; not so much in formulating rules of conduct as in considering what basis there can be for them.

The ethics built into the WMA guidelines are of universal application for sports medicine. So far as can be traced, they have never before been particularized and delineated in detail within a legal framework.

Furthermore, following the gross transgression of medical ethics during the Second World War, the World Medical Association (founded largely at the instigation of the BMA) restated the Hippocratic Oath in a modern style, this being known as the *Declaration of Geneva*. Upon this, an *International Code of Medical Ethics* was based.

## DECLARATION OF GENEVA

At the time of being admitted as a Member of the Medical
Profession I solemnly pledge myself to consecrate my life to the
service of humanity.
I will give to my teachers the respect and gratitude which is their
due;
I will practise my profession with conscience and dignity;
The health of my patient will be my first consideration;
I will respect the secrets which are confided in me;
I will maintain by all the means in my power the honour and the
noble traditions of the medical profession;
My colleagues will be my brothers;
I will not permit considerations of religion, nationality, race, party
politics or social standing to intervene between my duty and my
patient;
I will maintain the utmost respect for human life from the time of
conception; even under threat, I will not use my medical knowl-
edge contrary to the laws of humanity.
I make these promises solemnly, freely and upon my honour.

They are also consistent with the English text of the *International
Code of Medical Ethics* as follows:

*Duties of doctors in general*
A doctor *must* always maintain the highest standards of professional
conduct.
A doctor *must* practise his profession uninfluenced by motives of
profit.
The following practices are deemed unethical:
1.   Any self-advertisement except such as is expressly authorized by
the national code of medical ethics.
2.   Collaboration in any form of medical service in which the doctor
does not have professional independence.
3.   Receiving any money in connection with services rendered to a
patient other than a proper professional fee, even with the
knowledge of the patient.
Any act or advice which could weaken physical or mental resistance
of a human being may be used only in his interest.
A doctor is *advised* to use great caution in divulging discoveries or
new techniques or treatment.
A doctor *should* certify or testify only to that which he has
personally verified.

*Duties of doctors to the sick*
A doctor *must* always bear in mind the obligation of preserving
human life.
A doctor *owes* to his patient complete loyalty and all the resources

of his science. Whenever an examination or treatment is beyond his capacity he should summon another doctor who has the necessary ability.

A doctor *shall* preserve absolute secrecy on all he knows about his patient because of the confidence entrusted in him.

A doctor *must* give emergency care as a humanitarian duty unless he is assured that others are willing and able to give such care.

*Duties of doctors to each other*
A doctor *ought* to behave to his colleagues as he would have them behave to him.

A doctor *must not* entice patients from his colleagues.

A doctor *must* observe the principles of the Declaration of Geneva approved by the WMA.

This re-statement of Medical Ethics in modern style, with its universal application transcending Sports Medicine, can create understandable differing distillations of it at different points of the global compass. Within Britain, however, the BMA's *Sport and exercise medicine: policy and provision* (1996) publication (p. 10 *supra*) acknowledged its section headed 'Ethical considerations' to be based 'on the BMA's standard ethical guidance' (1993) (p. 8 *supra*) and concluded with the WMA declaration guidelines, reproduced in *its* Appendix 1 (see *here* Appendix II).

In that same year, 1993, Britain's General Medical Council (GMC) Education Committee, pursuant to its S. 5 Medical Act, 1983, obligations, published *Recommendations on Undergraduate Medical Education*, with a populist title *Tomorrow's Doctors*.

Five years later during these pages' gestation, a group of teachers of medical ethics and law in medical schools throughout the UK created a consultation paper for teaching undergraduates a core curriculum of medical ethics, consistent in principle with the WMA Guidelines since 1981.

Either through design or unawareness, the WMA Guidelines were ignored. Furthermore, there was no acknowledgement at all of medical undergraduates' sporting heritage, epitomized by the oldest rugby club in existence at Guy's Hospital, London, and one of the founder members of the Rugby Football Union in 1871. It was also the first club to have won the Hospitals Cup in 1875, a trophy for which London teaching hospitals have been competing annually since that first victory in 1875.

If there is a more effective way of *introducing* medical under-graduates to medical ethics than through sport and the WMA Guidelines it would be salutary to be aware of it. Furthermore, when the *Bulletin of Medical Ethics* in May 1998 commented on the proposed core curriculum it concluded:

The interests of the community are so little served by failing to educate doctors about medical ethics and the law that it is perhaps time that the GMC education committee had a majority of non-doctors as members.

Certainly those who participate in competitive and Corinthian sport upholding the Rule of Law generally would be suitable candidates.

**Table 1.1**

**List of UK sports activities which qualify for exemption as non-profit-making activities for VAT purposes, which inevitably require different and differing medical services. [HM Customs and Excise VAT 701/45/94]**

| | | |
|---|---|---|
| Aikido | Gymnastics | Real tennis |
| American football | Handball | Roller hockey |
| Angling | Hang/para gliding | Roller skating |
| Archery | Highland games | Rounders |
| Arm wrestling | Hockey | Rowing |
| Association football | Horse racing | Rugby League |
| Athletics | Hovering | Rugby Union |
| Badminton | Hurling | Sailing/yachting |
| Ballooning | Ice hockey | Sand/land yachting |
| Baseball | Ice skating | Shinty |
| Basketball | Jet skiing | Shooting |
| Baton twirling | Ju jitsu | Skateboarding |
| Biathlon | Judo | Skiing |
| Bicycle polo | Kabaddi | Skipping |
| Billiards | Karate | Snooker |
| Bobsleigh | Kendo | Snowboarding |
| Boccia | Korfball | Softball |
| Bowls | Lacrosse | Sumo wrestling |
| Boxing | Lawn tennis | Squash |
| Camogie | Life saving | Street hockey |
| Canoeing | Luge | Sub-aqua |
| Caving | Modern pentathlon | Surf life saving |
| Chinese martial arts | Motor cycling | Surfing |
| Cricket | Motor sports | Swimming |
| Croquet | Mountaineering | Table tennis |
| Crossbow | Movement and dance | Taekwondo |
| Curling | Netball | Tang soo do |
| Cycling | Orienteering | Tenpin bowling |
| Dragon boat racing | Parachuting | Trampolining |
| Equestrian | Petanque | Triathlon |
| Exercise and Fitness | Polo | Tug of war |
| Fencing | Pony trekking | Unihoc |
| Field sports | Pool | Volleyball |
| Fives | Quoits | Water skiing |
| Flying | Racketball | Weightlifting |
| Gaelic football | Rackets | Wrestling |
| Gliding | Racquetball | Yoga |
| Golf | Rambling | |

Chapter 1

# Sport and the law in the world of medicine

The international interaction between the worlds of sport, medicine and the law, with their respective global dimensions, should be self-evident to all who pause and reflect on their connections. For each discipline, Professor Ayer's concept of ethics as 'not so much ... formulating rules of conduct as ... considering what basis there can be for them' (see p. 16), is equally applicable. Thus, during a House of Lords debate on *Society's Moral and Spiritual Well-being* on the eve of the European Football competition in July 1996, Arsenal Football Club's most celebrated supporter, Dr George Carey, Archbishop of Canterbury, explained:

> We take it for granted that you cannot play a game of football without rules. Rules do not get in the way of the game; they make it possible.

For rules, lead Laws and the corollary can be seen in an editorial and board member of the American *The Physician and Sports Medicine*, Dr William O. Roberts in the May 1998 issue (Vol. 26, no. 5, p. 35: with my emphasis):

> The rules of the game are the fundamental primary strategy for preventing injury. They define standards of conduct for all players and allow them to expect certain responses. *Strict rule enforcement is critical to safety.* (Under the title *Keeping Sport Safe*.)

Without the laws of play and sanctions for enforcement there can be no true sport; and without identifiable and recognizable codes of conduct for medical, paramedical and associated practices there can be no consistent basis for administering to the health of participants and preventing abuses of sporting activities either on or off the 'fields of play'. Contrary to the wishes or beliefs of many who take part in sport, and also of many of those outside it, the law of the land does not stop at the touchline, boundary, board room or committee room.

Thus, medical ethics and the law within sport converge, to reflect the moral climate of civilized society as distinct from the jungle laws of commerce. Arguably with little difference, the FIMS *Code of Ethics in Sports Medicine* concludes:

> When speaking of ethics in sports medicine, one is not concerned with etiquette or law, but with basic morality.

Indeed, a recent publication of *An Intelligent Person's Guide to Ethics* from a former fellow and tutor in philosophy at St Hugh's College, Oxford, Baroness Warnock, states in the Introduction (1998):

> Ethics is a complicated matter. It is partly a matter of general principles, or even rules, like those of manners; but largely a matter of judgment and decision, of reasoning and sentiment, of having the right feeling at the right time, and every time is different. Above all it is a matter of trying to be a particular sort of person. And though ethics (or moral philosophy, as I prefer to call it), like the rest of philosophy has been secularised, it is almost impossible to think about the origins and development of morality itself without thinking about its interconnections with religion.

For those who still think the Ten Commandments even in a secularized society to be a sufficiently clear guide to ethical standards for a civilized society, and even for those who do not, the World Medical Association 'ethical guidelines for physicians in order to meet the needs of sportsmen or athletes . . .' provide a lead and fill a gap and need in a rapidly developing and complicated medical world.

Beyond this, the rapidity with which scientific experiments extend traditional treatment frontiers dictates a need for constant ethical vigilance and a continuing debate between medicine and the society it seeks to serve – as, for example, in the attitudes towards abortion, euthanasia, infertility, maintaining life in a persistent vegetative state, and prenatal surrogacy. For sports medicine, however, the WMA ethical guidelines have a global application, consistent with general medical ethical standards and accepted legal principles throughout the civilized world.

Variations in legal principles between nations are inevitable; and in the context of sports medicine it must be assumed that the practitioner will have qualified in and be familiar with his or her professional criteria and national codes of conduct. For sports medicine, however, the law operates in a unique and special way – a fact not always recognized within the legal profession.

For example, when a High Court judge (Curtis J) and the Court of Appeal established liability in negligence of an under-19 colts rugby referee for failing to understand and apply the laws of Rugby Union football (resulting in a collapsed scrum and paralysis of a schoolboy) (*Smoldon v Whitworth and Nolan* (1996) *Times,*

18 December), a solicitor, who had been a government-appointed Law Commissioner, complained in the *Solicitors Journal* (1996) 7 June, vol. 140, p. 550 of the unreasonableness of the decision (which had been welcomed medically by all fair minded rugby players and by other lawyers practising in this area). An international rugby player who was also a practising solicitor further complained about the decision in *Rugby World* (June 1996, p. 40).

The day before that referee's civil liability hearing ended, the Court of Appeal Criminal Division upheld nine months' custodial sentence of a Gloucester player who had smashed the jaw of a Rosslyn Park opponent and was found guilty of having caused serious bodily harm (*R v Devereux* (1996) *Times*, 26 February). On that occasion, too, complaints had been made about the justice of the decision, and even the decision to prosecute. Similar attitudes were aired when an international soccer player, Duncan Ferguson, was convicted and sentenced to imprisonment for head-butting an opponent during the course of a Scottish Premier League match (*Herald*, 25 May, 1995). This trend was confirmed when David Sole, the former Scottish rugby international captain, was reported as having written to a Scottish court supporting a fellow player, Jason Fayers (*Times*, 14 February, 1997) who had been fined £1000 and ordered to pay £500 compensation for breaking an opponent's jaw during a game. Earlier, he had been subjected by the Scottish Rugby Union to a four-year worldwide ban against participating in rugby in any format or role, concurrent with his court sentence. Thus, sport (within the UK at least) has moved forwards, in the eyes of the law, during the thirty years since the great international footballer Pele was brutally assaulted out of the 1966 football World Cup on English playing fields without any retaliation or sanction by the world governing body, FIFA, or in the criminal or civil courts. Nevertheless, during the summer of 1997, the expulsion of the Scottish rugby international Doddie Weir from the British Lions South African tour due to unprovoked foul play proved the perpetuation of this tendency. In the beginning of 1998, the rugby, legal and medical worlds were divided over the six month's suspension of a player following the finding that an opponent's ear had been bitten in a scrum. Later in 1998 towards commencement of the soccer World Cup competition, football was correspondingly divided over FIFA's direction, to referees for outlawing the potentially violent and *injurious* tackle from behind on an opponent by requiring the penal policy of a red card.

Accordingly, there is a culture gap between sport and society, which cannot be emphasized too often for sections of the sporting fraternity and even some members of the legal profession (at least in the UK). More particularly, it should not be overlooked that the law does not stop at the touchline or the boundary. This culture gap is compounded within sport itself – while the understandable and sustained attempts to eliminate cheating by drug abuse are consistent with the presentation and prevention of damage to health, comparable complaints about cheating by violence are conspicuous by their absence. Several legal levels may be identified for all sporting perspectives. These are set out below.

## THE LAW GENERALLY

The law in relation to sport operates at various levels, which are identifiable in the following way.

1   Playing laws:

   (a)   rules of play;

   (b)   sanctions and penalties for playing field offences (e.g. sending off, dismissals from play);

   (c)   disciplinary sanctions and penalties (e.g. suspensions and/ or fines).

2   National law:

   (a)   civil;

   (b)   criminal.

3   Consequences for breaches:

   (a)   playing laws – as above, suspension and/or fines;

   (b)   national laws – imprisonment, damages and compensation, each in accordance with the rules of national justice (i.e. knowledge of the precise accusation and admissible and effective evidence and an opportunity to challenge it, with or without evidence).

Referees and umpires control competitive sporting action within the playing legislative framework. They also have a duty of care for foreseeable risk to seriously injured participants, especially when regulating intended treatment by doctors. Breach of such duty by refusing a doctor's urgent access to the patient can create liability in negligence by referees and umpires, as in the distinguishing and special circumstances of *Smoldon v Whitworth and Nolan* (p. 22), when the referee failed to apply the modified Laws of the Game properly for an Under-19 Colts match. Furthermore, the frequent collision which exists between emotions and such intellectual energy as is left over from playing games surfaced when Ebsworth J injuncted the Welsh Rugby Union for failure to administer a fair disciplinary hearing to a player who had been sent off by a referee for unfair play, in breach of the laws of the game (*Jones v WRU, Times*, 6 March, 1997). Many lawyers, as well as administrators in the rugby world, failed to recognize the fundamental difference between the referee's sanction and the dismissal from further play and thereafter a fair hearing in the council chamber. Furthermore, when such a result has been achieved it is often hailed as a messianic revelation, without an awareness that in the United Kingdom sporting governing bodies have been biting the dust in court for more than 40 years, since the British Amateur Weightlifting Association was answerable to a complaining member before a High Court judge for a procedural irregularity (*Baker v Jones* (1954) I A.E.R. 553).

*Playing laws*

RULES OF PLAY

Sports medical and paramedical practitioners should familiarize themselves with each appropriate playing law for treatment on the playing area. The advice to doctors is that they should be familiar with both the laws of play and their entitlement to enter the playing arena for the purpose of treating injured players. Thus, concussion injuries demand mandatory ejectment from playing participation in rugby union football and professional horse-riding. Cricket umpires now have an onerous discretion to warn against unfair and dangerous play; and a doctor's capacity to advise and be activated by a boxing referee is easily recognizable. A ringside doctor advised the referee in July 1998 to stop Christopher Ewbank's World Heavyweight fight against Clive Thompson when his damaged eye unbalanced the fairness of the contest and this recalled the graphic criticism nearly a decade earlier of the celebrated critic and sympathizer with the fight game, Hugh McIlvanney, in the London *Observer* during November 1989, when Jim McDonnell's badly injured right eye led to:

> A series of misjudgements that could only provide encouragement for the abolitionist lobby. First, the referee, Joe Cortez, looked diligently into the sightless right eye and declined to intervene ... From his home in New Jersey last week, Cortez said the doctor merely advised him to 'watch the eye' (ignoring it would have been some feat) and did not recommend that the fight should be stopped.
> I find such a feeble response from the doctor incomprehensible,

until the ultimate intervention when the fight was stopped.

PENALTIES FOR OFFENCES

Again, sports medicine professionals should familiarize themselves with the sanctions for *any* breaches of playing laws for treatment on playing area, subject to the necessity for urgent access as above.

### *National Law: consequences for breaches*

CRIMINAL

Injuries caused by reckless and/or deliberate violent foul play create breaches of national as well as playing laws – a concept which has stood the test of time, since the first UK football field fatality in 1878 at Ashby-de-la-Zouch in Leicestershire. It lead to a criminal prosecution for murder (*R v Bradshaw* (1878) 14 Cox CC 83), followed by another in 1898 (*R v Moore* (1898) 14 TLR 229), with an endorsement as relatively recently as 1975 in the Court of Appeal (*R v Venna* [1975] 3 All ER 788): '*R v Bradshaw* ... can be read as supporting the view that unlawful, physical force applied recklessly constitutes a criminal offence.' Adverse comments on the efficacy and authenticity of these authoritative decisions in the criminal law in relation to sporting injuries have not diminished their enforceability.

CIVIL

The financial sanctions applied by the civil courts for breaches of playing law are consistent with those for medico-legal misconduct. Compensation for negligence or assault arising from the tort of trespass to the person, and the medical evidence of injuries are formidable weapons, and can be conclusive in establishing ultimate legal liability.

## SPORTS-RELATED MEDICO-LEGAL ISSUES

Medico-criminally, civil liability and legal issues reflect a general application not exclusive to sport. The sports medical world at every level is part of a wider canvas within which the categories of legal liability are never closed. Medico-legal jurisprudence is a dynamically developing subject, which transcends sports medicine. However, the traditional medico-legal texts rarely touch on sports medicine at least in the United Kingdom to date, although the USA and Canada, with their wider geographical and demographic areas alongside a litigation led culture provide vivid illustrations of liability, as these pages will show, with an oft-cited Canadian case of *Robitaille v Vancouver Hockey Club Ltd* ([1981] DLR 3rd 288) (vicarious liability through medical neglect by the medical staff of the Vancouver Ice Hockey Club, the Canucks), providing a valuable example (see p. 31).

The usual common law criteria for negligence (of a duty of care with a foreseeable risk of injury and breach causing damage to health with economic consequences) are no less applicable to all sports medicine activities, as they are to the traditional medico and paramedical and pharmacological legal areas, with variations for evidentiary requirements and the application of McNair J's classic test in *Bolam v Friern Barnet Hospital Management Committee* [1957] 1 WLR 582 at 587. It was applied and re-affirmed by the House of Lords with an emphasis on the levels of logical evidence and causation required in *Bolitho v City and Hackney H.A.* [1997] 4 AER 771 citing at 776b 'a doctor is not guilty of negligence if he has acted in accordance with a practice accepted as proper by a responsible body of medical men skilled in that particular art ... Putting it the other way round, a doctor is not negligent, if he is acting in accordance with such a practice, merely because there is a body of opinion that takes a contrary view.'

In Australia, however, a decision of the High Court upholding its appellate and New South Wales courts in *Rogers v Whittaker* [1992] 109 ALR 625 [1992] 4 MedL.R.79 (HC of Aust) with the robustness characteristic of its sporting culture has rejected the English Court's traditional deference to medical opinions epitomized in *Bolam* and *Bolitho*, and asserted the decision of the court itself as a matter of law in adjudicating whether a defendant's conduct has conformed to the standard of reasonable care demanded by the law, and not by the standard of the medical profession or some part of it.

A practical applicability of the Bolam formula for the sports medicine general practitioner is most conveniently and graphically illustrated by one of Britain's most experienced and respected lawyers, Sir James Comyn, who, after retiring from the judiciary, published a number of valuable reminiscatory volumes. As Domhnall McCauley has explained in a *British Journal of Sports Medicine* Editorial (June 1997, vol. 31, p. 91), 'Sports injury primary care in the United Kingdom is usually provided by general practitioners (GPs)'. In that context, Sir James Comyn's recollection from his memories in *Watching Brief* (1993) should be considered in conjunction with the Bolam criteria.

*The general practitioner*

A widow came to see me in consultation whose husband had recently died from malaria. The question was, could she sue the local medical doctor for negligence in failing to diagnose the illness – which would almost certainly have avoided the death of this otherwise fit 65-year-old man.

The doctor was the local general practitioner for an area based on a small village in the English midlands, about twenty years in practice. The deceased visited him on one occasion only, at visiting time. He told him that he had just returned from central Africa after a spell of duty, that he felt very unwell and that in particular he suffered from alternating chills and fever.

The doctor examined him, said he could find nothing the matter and that it was probably all due to the change of climate. He was prescribed a bottle of pick-me-up and told to come back in a week if there was no improvement. By the weekend the deceased was in hospital, diagnosed there and sent on to a tropical disease hospital where, although everything was done for him, he finally died.

We had no expert witnesses. I advised that we should at least find out whom to approach. I would like them in particular to say (a) whether an ordinary country GP should have diagnosed the trouble; (b) whether a week's delay would have made any difference; (c) whether the delay caused or contributed to the death; (d) whether the deceased's own delay of two days – before going to the doctor – facilitated the fatality; and (e) what the doctor should have done.

I reminded the client's solicitor that the doctor would have a union and experts acting for him and that until I saw, and if necessary cross-questioned them, I would not be able to express an opinion. I said that I felt particularly anxious about consulting a GP in the first place, and secondly about the short time-lag.

I received specialist reports within three weeks – both from experts in tropical diseases and both completely re-assuring. I had them to a consultation and they were united in their views.

They said that on the history given (central Africa, chills and fevers) any doctor should have diagnosed or suggested malaria and should have arranged his immediate admission into a tropical diseases or similar hospital. Any delay was potentially fatal; the extra delay caused or contributed to the death. The deceased's own delay of two days before going to the doctor was unfortunate but altered nothing.

As one said, 'This was a touch-and-go case and the doctor put it beyond repair.'

'Is it too much to expect the local GP to make an on-the-spot diagnosis of malaria?'

'Certainly not. It is one of the first subjects taught – in other words, the easiest one learns about.'

'Should not the deceased,' I asked, 'have suspected this himself with his African knowledge?'

'He might have suspected it but there are lots of other similar things – which a layman might think of. And anyway there is no evidence that he had ever had malaria before or been in touch with any case of it.'

We accordingly went ahead with the proceedings. They came before the late Mr Justice Cusack. Contrary to my expectations the other side called only the doctor (a very nice man) and a general consultant physician. The doctor deeply regretted what he said was his only wrong diagnosis. He knew about malaria but it never crossed his mind. He disputed the consequences on the ground I had always feared, the shortness of time.

The consultant acknowledged that the GP should have diagnosed or suspected malaria, but denied the consequences and said that it had already a fatal hold of the deceased and could not have been stopped. In the result the judge unhesitatingly accepted the widow's case and awarded her £10 000 and costs. The evidence of our experts was so overwhelming that there was no question of an appeal.

Against that introductory background, the sources which I have already written under the chapter title of '*Sports Medicine and the Law*' in *Sport and the Law* (Butterworths), and based upon *Mason and McCall Smith's Law and Medical Ethics*, are the basis for what follows, extended by identification of three additional categories in the context of (1) accident and emergency, (2) comparison with occupational health practitioners, (3) the Good Samaritan volunteers.

Primarily, categories of sports medical liability are based on the tort of negligence with its never too often repeated requirements to prove fivefold: (1) a duty of care; (2) a foreseeable risk of injury; (3) for which a breach; (4) causing injury; (5) creates compensatory damages awards.

In addition to the tort of negligence, liability can also arise (1) contractually and (2), in relatively rare cases, criminally.

1   While an Ontario Court in the Canadian case of *Pittman Estate v Bain* (1994) 112 DLR (4th) 257 has accepted the validity of a hospital–patient contractual relationship, the United Kingdom Common Law trend now leans away from a concurrent contract–tort liability relationship, although an argument has been floated that the Supply of Goods and Services Act 1982, ss. 4 and 9, could create a *statutory* contractual term for the fitness and quality of goods, if bodily products such as blood or semen are within its jurisdiction (see *Medical Negligence: Jones* 1996: p. 26 at Para. 2-013).

2   An express warranty was illustrated in another Canadian case of *La Fleur v Cornelis* (1979) 28 NBR (2d) 569 NBSC, where a

plastic surgeon universally told his patients 'There will be no problem, you will be very happy'. The subsequent scarring and deformity of one patient's nose did not create happiness or avoidance of liability, based upon breach of an express warranty, and creating a contractual liability.

Thus, the categories identified by Mason and McCall-Smith (1994, 4th edn) can now be delineated:

(a) vicarious liability;

(b) the reasonably skilful doctor: the usual practice: the custom test;

(c) misdiagnosis;

(e) the problem of the novice;

(f) protecting patients from themselves;

(g) *res ipsa loquitur*;

(h) injuries caused by drugs.

This raises the question of whether they can be applied to sport and to sports medicine in particular. The answer is: of course they can. The legal principle underlying every aspect of negligence with its duty of care–breach–foreseeability–causing–damage structure is constant for every different set of circumstances. All that sport does, as in every situation where the legal requirements appear for the first time, is to create a new level of awareness of how the general law applies to sports medicine within the framework of the WMA guidelines considered throughout these pages.

*Vicarious liability*

The solely legal issues involved in vicarious liability and sport, and the antithesis between general culpability and exclusion of liability for negligence (both general and medical) emerged dramatically in the 1958 Munich air disaster, which involved the famous 'Busby babes' and officials travelling with the Manchester United football team. The conflict of liability causation between ice on the wings and slush on the runway, dragged on for years until settled out of court. The vicarious liability was contested between whether the *airport* and/or the *aircraft* authorities were ultimately responsible in law for their officials' contribution to one of sport's most tragic disasters. The legal dispute's bitterness contrasted with the response of the staff at the Munich hospital where Sir Matt Busby and his fellow victims were admitted, whose medical skills and care in conditions of acute emergency earned universal acclaim and admiration.

That disaster illuminated the overlapping legal areas resulting from the expansion of international sport and the higher frequency of travel. In the UK, vicarious liability for medical negligence at hospital level had suffered from near immunity because of the frequent charitable elements involved in funding hospitals: see *Roe v Minister of Health, Woolley v Minister of Health* [1954] 2 QB 66, [1954] 2 All ER 131; *Razzall v Snowball* [1954] 3 All ER 429; *Higgins v North West Metropolitan Regional Hospital Board* [1955] 1 All ER 414. Following those cases, administrative arrangements were made between the various medical defence societies and the appropriate government departments for apportionment of damages awarded and costs, but since January 1990 the entire costs of negligence litigation are borne by the National Health Service (see, generally, Mason and McCall-Smith, 1994, 4th edn, 197).

Within that context, the front-line practitioners in the fight for fitness after treatment on the playing fields, at the ringside, or in the dressing room, are the accident and emergency department practitioners. They too, are subject to the 'duty of care' requirement, as appropriate to their training and experience. In areas of uncertainty or lack of expertise they should be prepared to consult a more experienced colleague and also to contact a patient's regular practitioner.

An example of the 'vicarious liability' principle in non-hospital medical malpractice emerges vividly from the facts in *Robitaille v Vancouver Hockey Club Ltd* [1981] DLR (3rd) 288 and the awards made by the British Columbia Court of Appeal in that case when it upheld the trial judge's damages award on a claim by a 28-year-old Canadian professional ice-hockey player, Mike Robitaille, against his former employer, the Vancouver Hockey Club known as the 'Canucks'. The basis for the decision turned upon the controlling links between the club and its doctor through the provision of car parking and ticket facilities in spite of there being no direct contractual relationship.

Sustained complaints to various club officials and doctors of injuries suffered in play were rejected in what was found by the judge to be an arrogant and high-handed manner. The neglect that was proved had resulted in considerable personal and professional losses and suffering. To establish a relationship involving vicarious liability it was necessary to determine the nature of the link between the doctor and the club. The level of control and involvement comprised a relatively modest bonus of $2500, season tickets, free parking, and access to the club lounge. The Canadian appeal court upheld the evidential findings of the trial judge (who had cited *Morren v Swinton and Pendelbury Borough Council* ([1965] 2 All ER 349 at 351) that:

> ... the measure of control asserted by the defendant over the doctors in carrying out their work was substantial. The degree of control need not be complete in order to establish vicarious liability. In the case of a professional person, the absence of control and direction over the manner of doing the work is of little significance.

Also confirmed were the trial judge's damages awards:

(a)   $175 000 for loss of professional hockey income;

(b)   $85 000 for loss of future income other than from professional hockey;

(c)   $40 000 for pain, suffering and loss of enjoyment of life.

Of equal significance for all sportspersons was a concurrent approval by the appeal court of the trial judge's conclusion about the plaintiff's contributory negligence. He was held to be:

> 20% at fault because his failure to take any action [i.e. to complain] to protect his own interest was less than reasonable. There was evidence upon which Esson J could find that Robitaille was negligent ... the trial judge correctly distinguished cases ... which dealt with factory workers ... dealing here with a highly paid experienced modern day professional athlete and not a factory worker responding to the mores of olden times. The court's assessment of the plaintiff's contributory negligence (due to his not pursuing his medical complaints with agencies outside the negligent club's control earlier than he did) was possibly harsh. Nevertheless, the trial judge heard extensive oral evidence, and his final awards, which included aggravated and exemplary damages, demonstrated his ultimate awareness of the plaintiff's overriding and justifiable grievance about medical neglect, which created the clear-cut vicarious liability.

This case should be contrasted with *Wilson v Vancouver Hockey Club* (1983) 5 DLR (4n) 282, BC SC; affirmed 22 DLR (4n) 516, CA. The British Columbia Court of Appeal affirmed the trial judge's decision that the doctor in the case was an independent contractor on the facts of the case and the club was exonerated from liability, notwithstanding the club doctor's personal professional negligence upon a delayed diagnosis of cancer. This liability emerged because the evidence indicated that the doctor made his decision on treatment without the advice of the club management, and because the doctor felt he served the interests of the players exclusively and that his primary obligation was to them, acting as an independent contractor and not as a servant of the hockey club.

The earlier attitude of the Canucks' medical team towards Mike Robitaille spills over into associated territories, illustrated most conveniently by the awareness in American courts of a 'Good Samaritan' concept. The no-win-no-fee basis of much American litigation has resulted in legislative intervention, with nationwide 'Good Samaritan' statutes creating immunity from litigation for various kinds of negligence. The valuable section by Emidio A. Bianco and Elmer J. Walker, *Sports Medicine for the Primary Physician*, 2nd edition (1994), edited by Richard B. Birrer (see p. 95 below) setting out various categories of sport, explains at p. 28 how readers:

> ... should not preoccupy themselves with the distinction between ordinary and gross negligence other than to remember that any 'major' deviation from the standard of care, which is flavored by what appears to be a conscious or reckless disregard for the safety of another, might be considered 'gross negligence'. For example, a physician is aware that an injured athlete is sprawled on the playing field and has sustained a head injury, but nevertheless undertakes to treat before understanding the mechanisms of the injury, or before examining the athlete's head, neck and extremities. Immediately thereafter, the person becomes quadriplegic. The physician may be liable for gross negligence, because every physician is aware, or should be aware, that head injury may be associated with cervical spine injury, and that movement of the cervical spine in such cases may worsen a spinal cord injury (a clear and present danger).

Without invoking statutory intervention, the common law outside the USA has arrived at a similar conclusion, spanning 140 years, as two cases from different periods demonstrate.

1   In *Goode v Nash* (1979) 21 SASR 419, S.C. free glaucoma screenings were being performed, with an experienced general practitioner, Dr Goode, providing his services voluntarily. When he placed a hot tonometer upon the patient's left eye, a burn was suffered which left the patient with scaring of the cornea and reduced vision. A claim against Dr Goode for negligence succeeded because, although he was engaged in a valuable community service entirely on a voluntary basis, he was nevertheless liable to pay damages.

2   In *Gladwell v Steggel* (1839) 5 Bing, 733 8 LJCP 361 3 JUR 535, 8 Scott 60, a 10-year-old girl complained of a pain in her knee while walking in fields with her father. Her parents summoned

the defendant, a clergyman who 'also practised as a medical man', with disastrous consequences which entitled them to succeed from 'a breach of duty arising out of the employment of the Defendant by the Plaintiff'. This was an action *ex delicto*. As *Jackson* and *Powell* on *Professional Negligence* (1997) comment at p. 594 para b-07, with a footnote citing *Goode v Nash*:

> The medical practitioner assumes duty of care to the patient, even when he renders his services gratuitously or entirely voluntarily, for example by attending the venue of a road accident.

Consequently, the practitioner who intervenes outside his domain with an adverse result, even if acting *in extremis*, is likely to be found negligent.

### *The reasonably skilful doctor: the usual practice: the custom test*

The onward march of medicine towards new frontiers cannot be ignored. The names of Louis Pasteur, Madame Curie and Alexander Fleming are familiar to the layperson, and in sports medicine, too, there is a level of public awareness. Anyone with an interest in sport who remembers the 1950s will recall the public tension surrounding the fate of Mr Denis Compton's knee-cap. After initial consultations with W. E. (Bill) Tucker, based upon his mix of orthopaedic skills and international rugby playing experiences for England under the captaincy of Wavell Wakefield, it was extracted by Mr Osmond-Clarke, FRCS, thus allowing his patient to continue playing test and county cricket with much success. The knee-cap itself was kept as a memento by Tucker, who later presented it to the MCC, in whose archive it has since remained at Lord's, in a biscuit tin: a macabre slice of medico-sporting history memorabilia. Mr Compton had by then retired from an active professional footballing career, so the novelty of this form of surgery did not involve his return to that game. Nevertheless, the intervening years have witnessed a great reduction in the recovery period for such an operation; from the days when a conventional cartilage operation would incapacitate a footballer for weeks, to modern arthroscopic surgery, which can return a player to training within days.

Against this background of mobility in thinking and technology, what norm should be applied? Each specialist area of medicine has its own specialist knowledge with interdisciplinary connections. A trainer or physiotherapist/podiatrist would not necessarily be expected to have the same level of expertise as an experienced physician or surgeon (although in some areas of practice, certain skills will be greater in therapists).

There are three landmark House of Lords decisions on medical duties: *Sidaway v Board of Governors of the Bethlem Royal Hospital and Maudsley Hospital* [1985] AC 871, [1985] 1 All ER 643 (warning of risks) and *Maynard v West Midlands Regional Health Authority* [1985] 1 All ER 635, [1984] 1 WLR 634 (conflicting medical opinions) re-affirmed in *Bolitho* (at pp. xxv and 27 *supra*). Yet, on the basic issue of what is the usual or customary level of skill to apply, Lord Scarman reiterated long-established principles from the 1950s. In *Sidaway* ([1985] 1 All ER 643 at 649) he referred to a jury direction by McNair J in the leading case of *Bolam v Friern Hospital Management Committee* [1957] 2 All ER 188, [1957] 1 WLR 582:

> ... as a rule that a doctor is not negligent if he acts in accordance with a practice accepted at the time as proper by a responsible body of medical opinion even though other doctors adopt a different practice. In short, the law imposes a duty of care; but the standard of care is a matter of medical judgement.

In *Maynard* ([1985] 1 All ER 635 at 638) he said: 'I do not think that words of the Lord President (Clyde) in *Hunter v Hanley* [1955] SLT 213 and 217 can be bettered':

> 'In the realm of diagnosis there is ample scope for genuine difference of opinion and one man clearly is not negligent merely because his conclusion differs from that of other professional men ... The true test for establishing negligence in diagnosis or treatment on the part of a doctor is whether he has been proved to be guilty of failure as no doctor of ordinary skill would be guilty of acting with ordinary care. ...

and in *Bolitho* (p. 27 *supra*) Lord Browne-Wilkinson referred back to Lord Scarman in *Maynard* repeating in different words McNair's *Bolam* test.

*Misdiagnosis*

The potential danger for this category of negligence must be realized by all concerned with athletic injuries in every sport where judgments have to be made under pressures of time and circumstances (e.g. television cameras and a crowded arena). Mason and McCall-Smith (1994, 4th edn) explain:

A mistake in diagnosis will not be considered negligent if [the usual] standard of care [in dealing with patients] is observed but will be treated as one of the non-culpable and inevitable hazards of practice.

A footnote cites a judicial observation that:

Unfortunate as it was that there was a wrong diagnosis, it was one of those misadventures, one of those chances, that life holds for people (*Crivon v Barnet Group Hospital Management Committee* (1958) Times, 19 November).

However, Canada again provides a direct example of liability, which was established this time in the Ontario Court of Appeal (*Price v Milawski, Murray and Castroyan* (1978) 82 DLR (3d) 130). A 41-year-old tool and dye worker broke his right *ankle* when playing soccer with his young son. A negligently erroneous X-ray prescription for attention to the right *foot* was compounded by a cascade of consequential errors involving more than one medical practitioner who successively consolidated earlier misdiagnosis. This resulted in a Canadian appellate court's confirmation of the trial judge's ruling that 'one negligent doctor could be liable for the additional loss caused by the other'. The appeal court also upheld the damages award of $50 000 for the general damages, which included $34 465 for loss of income up to the date of trial. The successive misdiagnoses proved very expensive for the doctors, who included a radiologist, as well as painful for the patient.

Another misdiagnosis of an ankle injury appears in a case note contained in Powers and Harris (1990), p. 666, para 30-28. While playing squash, a 40-year-old regular male player suddenly felt severe pain on the back of the ankle, 'as if a brick had been thrown at me and I fell to the ground'. The hospital doctor failed to make a correct diagnosis of a ruptured achilles tendon, assessing simply ruptured fibres which required no treatment. Two days later, the general practitioner ordered physiotherapy without examination. Two months later, an orthopaedic surgeon made the correct diagnosis and complicated reconstructive surgery was required. The commentary that prompt diagnosis and treatment would have prevented disability also pointed to an indefensible position and that the history was typical of a ruptured achilles tendon, for which clinical examination is only necessary to confirm the diagnosis.

## Negligence in treatment

The examples above illustrate negligence in treatment. A grey area exists between negligence and error of judgment, as illuminated by *Whitehouse v Jordan* [1981] 1 All ER 267, [1981] 1 WLR 246, in which a baby was pulled too hard with forceps with resulting asphyxia and brain damage. The House of Lords refined Lord Denning's distinction between negligence and error of judgment when the trial judge's damages award of £100 000 was overturned on the basis that he drew the wrong inferences of fact from the oral and documentary evidence. In the House of Lords, Lord Fraser explained ([1981] 1 All ER 267 at 281):

> The true position ... depends on the nature of the error. If it is one that would not have been made by a reasonably competent professional man professing to have the standard and type of skill that the defendant holds himself out as having, and acting with ordinary care, then it is negligence. If, on the other hand, it is an error that such a man, acting with ordinary care, might have made, then it is non-negligent.

In *Whitehouse v Jordan* a conflict of medical testimony caused the Court of Appeal and the House of Lords to adjudicate that the very experienced trial judge had drawn the wrong inferences of fact from the conflicting medical evidence. In sports medicine, as a developing science and discipline, the possibility of conflict between genuine specialist opinions can inevitably exist, a state of affairs which often develops when tensions arise between medical advisers and sports physiotherapists of comparable if not greater experience, but lesser qualifications.

### The problem of the novice

Every professional is at first an amateur. The beginner must be guided by instructions. The criteria laid down by the House of Lords (see *Sidaway*, p. 35) 'accepted at the time as proper by a reasonable body of medical opinion' conditions the standards appropriate to the different levels of medical or paramedic activity. Thus, an important unreported case, *Cattley v St John's Ambulance Brigade* (1988), QBD (cited in Jones (1996) but not referred to generally in the recognized sources), explains how the standard of care required of a first aider is not that of a doctor but that of an ordinary skilled first aider, exercising and professing to have the special skill of a first aider. This is comparable to the fledgling athlete who is projected into action with veterans: public allowances of limited sympathy for youth alongside maturity will not include forgiveness for substandard performances. The law does not differentiate either. If liability arises, it could be vicarious for an employer or controller of a practitioner associated with medical services, whether as doctor, physiotherapist, podiatrist, trainer or traditional sponge man. The amateur club which permits an unqualified member to act as an *ad hoc* first aid assistant without any practical experience, resulting in any serious or actionable injury, is as much at risk as the hospital committee which allows an inexperienced practitioner to carry out complex operations usually reserved for expert staff: see *Brown v Lewis* (1896) 12 TLR 455 (Blackburn Rovers Football Club personal committee member's liability when negligent subcontracting caused liability).

*Protecting patients from themselves*

This particular category in the reported cases is concerned with suicide attempts and tendencies. An analogy can apply to excessively enthusiastic athletes who strive to return to action when not fully fit: in effect, a form of career suicide. Without firm medical guidance, emphasizing the harmful consequences of the zest for play overriding the consequences of such medical advice, then a liability for negligence could well arise.

The demands and stresses of competitive professional sport are particularly vulnerable in this category. With a supreme irony, unnoticed by many commentators at the time of the 1996–97 FA cup final, manager Bryan Robson selected, or allowed to be selected, a semi-fit player for the Middlesbrough team, Ravanelli, a quarter of a century after he was himself selected for the England 1970 World Cup tour in Mexico after suffering a dislocated shoulder while playing for Manchester United. This reflected a memorable comment during an interview on the BBC World Service during 1997 given by FIFA Secretary General, Seb Blatter 2–3 May, 1997 when questioned by Steve Tongue:

> It is always the best players that have to perform. It is too much to demand for every game. The clubs pay a lot for players. They have to make players like horses. They perform but they are not in a circus. They are in a game and they need time off for recuperation. Otherwise there are physical limits and there are mental limits to play a game.

Added to the demands of the club are the contractual pressures of sponsors and agents. No veterinary surgeon would allow horses to perform to the extent demanded of two-legged athletes: indeed, if such demands on animals were ever made, the RSPCA would become involved. It has often protested in the past, for example at the Grand National dangers, for protection of the horses, with a consequential benefit to the riders; and illustrative of the different approaches for four-legged from two-legged animals were the contrasting attitudes explained publicly during the high sporting summer of 1998. The Epsom Derby winner's trainer, Luca Cumani, was recorded in the *Sunday Times* (19 July) by John Karter, to say of his colt, High Rise:

> We bypassed the Irish Derby to run at Ascot for the King George VI and Queen Elizabeth Stakes because I have the Prix de l'Arc de Triomphe at the back of my mind and we wanted to save the horse for the autumn.

A week later Britain's women's heptathlon champion Denise Lewis wrote in the *Daily Mail* (24 July) under the headline 'Stop pushing our track stars to the point of collapse':

> Athletes' bodies are not machines. All the exertion takes its toll and it is hardly surprising a lot of us end up injured. Our bodies need 12 months without the pressure of a major championship to recharge.

At present, there is no Society for the Prevention of Cruelty to Human Athletes.

*Res ipsa loquitur*

This penultimate stage in Mason and McCall-Smith's classification of medical negligence has been the subject of both critical and literal commentaries in the House of Lords: see *Ballard v North British Railway Co* (1923) SC (HL) 43 at 46, where Lord Shaw of Dunfermline said: 'If that phrase had not been in Latin, nobody would have called it a principle … The day for canonising Latin phrases has gone past.' Denning LJ (as he then was) brought it all into focus in a hospital negligence case (*Cassidy v Ministry of Health* [1951] 2 KB 343 at 365, [1951] 1 All ER 574 at 588) with the judgment that the plaintiff in the case before him on appeal was entitled to say: 'I went into hospital to be cured of two stiff fingers. I have come out with four stiff fingers and my hand is useless. That should not have happened if due care had been used. Explain it if you can.' Lord Normand in *Barkway v South Wales Transport Co Ltd* [1950] 1 All ER 398 at 399 explained that it is:

> … no more than a rule of evidence affecting onus. It is based on common sense, and its purpose is to enable justice to be done when the

facts bearing on causation and on the care exercised by the defendant are at the outset unknown to the plaintiff and are or ought to be within the knowledge of the defendant.

More recently in *Ratcliffe v Plymouth & Torbay HA and Exeter & North Devon HA* 1998, PIQR P170, the trial judge and Court of Appeal re-affirmed the necessity for *prima facie* positive evidence to establish the principle, where an insufficiency of proof defeated a negligence claim based upon a spinal injection injury. In language appropriate to this context, Brooke LJ said at p. 176:

> Medical science is not all-knowing. The Greek tragedian Aeschylus addressed the unforeseen predicaments of human frailty in terms of the sport of the gods. In a modern scientific age, the wisest of experts will sometimes have to say:
> 'I simply do not know what happened.'
> The courts would be doing the practice of medicine a considerable disservice if in such a case, because a patient has suffered a grievous and unexpected outturn from a visit to a hospital, a careful doctor is ordered to pay him compensation as if he had been negligent in the care he afforded to his patient.

Finally, Canada provides one more graphic example which would have horrendous consequences for any athlete. The plaintiff entered hospital for treatment of a fractured ankle and left with an amputated leg. No explanation existed. The evidence, applying the principles cited above, pointed in one inevitable direction: negligence (*MacDonald v York County Hospital Corporation* [1972] 28 DLR 3d 521) (see also as failure to consult further: Chapter 6 'Guideline 5' at p. 91).

*Injuries caused by drugs*

Mason and McCall-Smith (1994), p. 213, explain in the broadest dimension how:

> The extensive use of drugs and other medical products in modern medical practice, coupled with the wide variety of available substances and devices, inevitably leads to a high incident of injuries for which they are responsible;

and in the sporting context a valuable contribution from a section on 'Therapeutic drugs', in the *Clinics in Sports Medicine Series* volume on *Sports Pharmacology* during July 1998, from John M. Henderson DOM FAAFP, at the Mercer University School of Medicine, Macon, Georgia, explained succinctly in summary form:

> Sports medicine is a reflection of the type and quality of medicine

practised in the community in general. In turn, the practice of medicine is a reflection of society, its cultural biases and mores. The use of medication in the treatment of athletes requires special consideration on the part of the physician so that the athlete is not put in a compromising condition or in jeopardy of disqualification. Periodic familiarity with the updated lists of banned substances, knowledge of the requisites of the particular sport, and, most importantly, knowledge of the athletes themselves will help minimize medication-related problems.

Nevertheless for sportspersons and sports medical practitioners, however, the social evil inherent in the drug trade raises legal, medical, ethical and sporting administrative issues which were crystallized by two leading sports personalities in a manner discussed below. This crucial social (as well as sporting) problem cannot be emphasized too strongly for sport. It is also one which extends beyond the level of medical injuries caused by incorrectly or negligently prescribed drugs, into the wider and equally significant career injuries suffered by the sports patient whose lawfully prescribed drug treatment conflicts with the rules of a sporting governing body. Furthermore, two West Sussex general practitioners, Peter and Mary Greenway in a paper for the BASM *British Journal of Sports Medicine* for June 1997 at p. 129 concluded that the responses to a questionnaire 'suggest that general practitioners [at least in the West Sussex area] need to be better informed of current and updated guidelines'. They ended with an unanswerable question: 'How this is best achieved is yet to be established'. One answer, confirmed for this author by Donald Macleod, is contained at the end of the valuable chapter on 'Drug misuse' from Dr David A. Cowan, director of the Drug Control and Teaching Centre at King's College, London in the *British Medical Journal*'s equally valuable *ABC of Sports Medicine*. He concluded at p. 56 'The *British National Formulary* now carries details of a helpline for doctors who need guidance about whether drugs they are offering to patients who also compete in sport might be banned from that sport' (see no. 35: March 1998, Appendix IV, p. 154 *infra*).

Two examples which are cited in this chapter (Ron Angus (from judo) and Willie Johnston (football)) *On the Wing*, not only identified a developing area which has yet to be thought through between the interlocking worlds of sport, medicine and the law, but also illuminate the revolution which has projected sport from a healthy, fun-loving, competitive and educative pastime into a ruthlessly commercialized and often corrupt sector of the entertainment industry, containing within it seeds of destruction for health and society generally in addition to sport. They raise questions for the future which have yet to be acknowledged and faced by sport and society for which an answer can be provided only in part by the law.

The foundation for the claim that 'an answer can be provided only in part by law' was confirmed at Doncaster on St Leger Day, Saturday 12 September, 1987. The Home Office announced that it had asked the Advisory Council on the Misuse of Drugs to consider whether steroids should be included in the Misuse of Drugs Act 1971. A bulletin entitled *Drugs in Sport, a Reappraisal* from the Institute of Medical Ethics claimed to raise two main questions:

1    Is it unethical for a sportsman to take drugs?

2    Is drug taking so serious a problem that the governing bodies of sports need to draw up rules to prevent it, with punishments for contravention of the rules?

The premise on which the questions were posed challenged the existence of these health hazards beyond sport (as identified by Donohue and Johnston (1986), or in Grant (1985)). Finally, Pacemaker International (1987) explained the dangers for the breeding side of horse racing, that Bute and Lasix, which are permitted under rules in most American states, 'may mask congenital deficiencies in horses that will later be passed on to their offspring, thus having a detrimental effect on the breed'. Indeed, in the context of this trespass upon nature it is pertinent to enquire whether two-legged animals are so very different from four-legged ones. This trio of publications proves the complexity of the subject and the need, in Britain at least, for an in-depth assessment based upon authentic evidence of the quality of both celebrated Reports to which Sir John Wolfenden gave his name, i.e. *Homosexuality and Prostitution* (1957) and *Sport and the Community* (1960).

## DRUGS

Any misconception that the current concern is a recent phenomenon can be dispelled by recalling the symposium mounted in 1985 by the Sports Council at King's College, London. It occurred when the Council's campaign for drug testing among sporting governing bodies was backed by a formidable body of oral, documentary and visual evidence. This explained graphically the adverse health consequences of rule-breaking by those indulging in drug-taking throughout the sporting world, both domestically and internationally. It was concerned primarily with the interrelationship between the health and ethical problems in sport. It was not concerned directly with the wider aspects of the conflict of laws in sport which are set out below.

In January 1984 the British Judo Association announced that a dope test on Ron Angus – winner of the under 78 kg category in the All England Championship in December 1983 – had proved positive. A sample contained traces of a stimulant, pseudo-Ephedrine (*Sunday Telegraph*, 4 January, 1984). Angus, who had dual Canadian-British nationality, claimed that the substance must have been contained in a sinus decongestant which he had taken under a lawful medical prescription by his Canadian doctor. Because he had breached the Association's requirements, he was banned for life from competing in British championships. Five months later, after he had taken legal advice, the High Court in London lifted the ban. It was admitted by the Association that the absence of a hearing in which Angus could explain his position breached the rules of natural justice, and the life ban was duly rescinded. The Association's rules have now been tightened to place the onus on competitors, and by implication, therefore, on their *personal doctors* to ensure that lawful medication does not contain banned substances (*Daily Telegraph*, 15 June, 1984).

Yet wider publicity was suffered by Scottish football international Willie Johnston, sent home from the 1978 FIFA World Cup. From the explanation in his book (*On the Wing*) and in the medico-legal opinion expressed at the Sports Council symposium, Johnston appears to have suffered an avoidable and gross injustice. His own *English* Football League club doctor had lawfully prescribed Reactivan pills for Johnson's nasal condition. The *Scottish* FA doctor had warned him about drugs; but Johnston had not realized that his pills contained the stimulant Fencamsamin, of which traces were found after a positive dope test, in breach of FIFA rules. Johnston's international football career was blighted without any apparent personal culpability on his part. No complaint was made to FIFA by anyone on Johnston's behalf, and the fact that FIFA's registered office is in Switzerland takes it outside the jurisdiction of the UK courts. Thus, Johnston could not *directly* have made a claim in Scotland against the disciplinary governing body, FIFA, similar to that successfully made by Ron Angus against the British Judo Association, unless he had emulated comparable claimants and sued his own Scottish FA. Yet, on the facts summarized above from Johnston's own account, he was almost certainly innocent of any offence under British criminal law. Indeed, s. 28(3)(b)(i) of the Misuse of Drugs Act 1971 provides that any accused person shall be acquitted of a drug offence 'if he proves that he neither believed nor suspected nor had reason to suspect that the substance or product in question was a controlled drug', i.e. one of which the use is controlled by the Act, and thereby unlawful generally. That subsection illustrates the problems which face sportsmen who require drugs lawfully for medicinal purpose; namely difficulties of accurate knowledge regarding allowable and non-allowable drugs and preparations:

1    How are athletes and their personal doctors to know when a breach or potential breach of the rules against drug abuse of a sports governing body occurs?

2    How are sports governing bodies to know that a failure to meet their own stringent rules for the protection of a particular sport does or does not arise from a lawful medicinal prescription?

And, with greater difficulty:

3    How are lawyers to balance the interest of the sport in which they advise administrators with the need to respect the rights of individual competitors?

4    What is the patient to do when faced with what may become a conflict of personal health interests against the undoubted right in a free society to participate in healthy competition?

These questions cannot be evaded, and have to be thought through within the framework of what lawyers recognize as a conflict of laws situation. Furthermore, with the expansion of international sport, and the recognition of the problem by the WHO, as well as international governing bodies, there is the added issue of international harmony when attempting to formulate solutions.

As sport becomes more commercially competitive and its television-regulated coverage increasingly global, the need to ensure that it is kept within a healthy framework demands a co-ordinated effort from everyone concerned, along the lines suggested below. Without such concord, recourse to the courts or some form of legal investigation is bound to follow.

1    *Doctors, physiotherapists and podiatrists* who treat patients competing athletically must familiarize themselves with the requirements of the particular sport in question – at both domestic and international level – and pass on this information to their patients.

2    *Lawyers* who advise administrators must ensure that any regulations to prevent cheating do not either transgress rules of natural justice (e.g. the opportunity to be heard), or contravene the spirit of the 'ignorance of the facts' defence in drugs cases.

3   *Administrators* should try, with doctors, pharmacists, lawyers and drug manufacturers, to attain a balance between a sport's rules and an individual's medicinal requirements, in the interests of fair play, health and the avoidance of cheating.

4   *Competitors* must familiarize themselves with their own medical requirements within the rules laid down by their particular sport.

The problem of the widespread use of steroids within sport was highlighted when Ben Johnson was caught using steroids in the 1988 Los Angeles Olympics and the legal floodgates opened shortly after Johnson's positive test for stanozolol, when the government of Canada appointed the Hon Charles L. Dubin to lead the '*Commission of inquiry into the use of drugs and banned practices intended to enhance athletic performance*'. This has been the most detailed and innovative report so far published on the subject. In the report, Dubin CL said of the problem that 'the evidence shows that banned performance-enhancing substances and in particular anabolic steroids are being used by athletes in almost every sport, most extensively in weightlifting and track and field'.

Robert Armstrong QC, a member of the Canadian Bar Association and Commission Counsel to the Dubin Inquiry, stated at an international symposium on sport and the law held in Monaco in 1991 that, in Seoul, Canada had lost its innocence as a sporting nation. The Dubin Inquiry showed that the use of drugs within sport had no national boundaries. Dr Robert Kerr, a doctor practising in San Gabriel, testified before the inquiry that he had prescribed anabolic steroids to approximately twenty medallists in the 1984 Olympics. At the US Senate Judiciary on steroid abuse, Pat Connolly, a coach of the women's track team, estimated that five out of ten gold medallists in the US men's Olympic track team used anabolic steroids at Seoul.

The most common forbidden performance-enhancing techniques are the use of steroids, human growth hormone and blood doping. Blood doping involves the athlete taking blood out of his or her own body and then re-injecting it several weeks later, a few days before the event, in order to increase their oxygen-carrying capacity, thereby improving performance. This is a sophisticated concept, used at higher levels of sport, and is not a problem generally encountered by the average GP practising sports medicine. These banned practices are apparently adopted by a significant number of athletes and only one deterrent exists: testing both in and out of competition.

Dope testing in Britain is governed by the Sports Council, which has an accredited IOC laboratory and which has implemented one of the most stringent programmes in the world. In 1992 over 4000 samples were taken from athletes in fifty-three different sports, with a higher number than ever before coming from testing out of competition. However, it is difficult to assess just how effective a deterrent dope testing is. Given that Ben Johnson was tested positive for a second time in March 1993 despite having suffered so much humiliation at the Seoul Olympics, it is clear that for some athletes it is *not* an effective enough deterrent. Furthermore, at the time of writing, Johnson's legal advisers were reported to be contemplating an appeal to the IAAF against a lifetime ban, on the basis of a restraint of trade plea.

The prohibited use of steroids within sport has resulted in much litigation in recent years. Many athletes challenge bans imposed on them after a positive test. For example, a 25-year-old Swiss athlete, Sandra Gasser, who had attained international standard in the 800 metres and the 1500 metres, appealed to the Chancery Division of the High Court after she was suspended for two years from eligibility to enter athletics competitions held under IAAF rules, following a positive test of the metabolite of methyl testosterone at the 1987 World Championships in Rome. An arbitration panel of the IAAF affirmed the decision (*Gasser v Stinson* (1988)).

Scott J refused declaratory relief by writ (rather than by the usual judicial review procedure) that the suspension was unreasonably in restraint of trade (although he accepted that the restraint of trade principles applied to the facts of the case) (15 June, 1988, unreported) *Sport and the Law* (1994), 2nd edn, Grayson, p. 304. More significantly, however, he made two observations suggesting a different approach by the plaintiff's lawyers might have had different consequences. First, he found relating to one of the two tested urine samples: 'The Panel might have found that the other explanation was too conjectural to be accepted. But no evidence to incline them to the view had been put before them by the plaintiff or the SLV.' Second, he explained that the panel:

> ... accepted the other explanation. They may have been wrong in doing so. They may have been wrong in regarding the identified procedural failure as not material. But unless they exceeded their jurisdiction, exceeded, that is to say, their terms of reference, the plaintiff is stuck with their conclusions. Any remedy of appeal to the High Court under the Arbitration Acts is long since time-barred.

Furthermore, Robert Armstrong QC, at the 1991 Monaco symposium said that 'basically, Dubin recommended that in order to have a fair right of appeal, athletes should be in a position to be able to test the scientific validity of the test results'. The question therefore remains, could different evidence in *Gasser v Stinson* have produced a different result?

Katrin Krabbe, the German athlete, successfully overturned one IAAF ban for drug abuse in 1993, and has challenged another ban imposed on her for the alleged use of the drug Clenbuterol. Andrew Saxton and Andrew Davies, the British weightlifters sent home from the 1992 Barcelona Olympics after being tested positive for Clenbuterol, have argued that their use of the substance did not justify disqualification as the drug was not on the IOC's list of banned substances at the time of competition.

The British sprinter, Jason Livingstone, was also sent home from the Barcelona Olympics as he was tested positive for the drug methandionanone in a random out-of-competition test before the Olympics. He appealed to the BAF Independent Appeals Panel, which dismissed his appeal by a 2-1 majority in May 1993. In the appeal, there was an attempt to cast doubt over the positive test because, in fact, a *metabolite* of methandianone had been found, not the actual substance. Livingstone argues that just because a metabolite of 6 beta-hydroxyl methandianone had been found, this was not conclusive proof that he had actually used methandianone. This view was based on the evidence of Professor Arnold Beckett, previously a member of the IOC's medical commission. However, the majority of the panel felt that the evidence which was before them put beyond reasonable doubt that Livingstone had taken the drug.

In December 1993, Harry ('Butch') Reynolds obtained judgment in a court in Ohio against the IAAF for damages for $27.3m for wrongfully banning him from athletics. Following a competition in Monaco in August 1990, Reynolds was randomly tested and it was found that he had traces of the anabolic steroid nandrolone in his urine. The IAAF did not seek to defend the proceedings and subsequently argued that the Ohio court had no jurisdiction over the IAAF and chose to ignore the judgment. It should be noted that the Ohio court accepted as correct everything that Reynolds said in his complaint, since the proceedings were not defended. The award of damages, therefore, was not a result of conclusions based on evidence heard from both sides on the merits of the case, and on an appeal to the Supreme Court, the judgment in favour of Reynolds was reversed.

Another contentious example to illustrate the problem emerged after a rugby international between France and Wales in Paris during 1992. Anthony Clement and Jean-Baptiste Lafond were allegedly tested positive for the use of prohibited drugs. In due course, it emerged that Malcolm Downes, the Welsh Rugby Union honorary surgeon had prescribed Clement drugs for sickness and dysentery. Lafond had been administered with Pholeodine for a cough by a French doctor. In due course each player was exonerated, but what emerged is that the Welsh Rugby Union uses the same list of banned substances as the IOC, which differs from the list adopted by the French Rugby Union.

Correspondingly, after an international conference of rugby doctors had recommended criteria for drug testing, the International Rugby Board needed reminding of the necessity of creating sanctions for positive test findings.

At the time of writing, two attempts were made in the High Court to invoke the assistance of the Treaty of Rome in circumventing sanctions imposed by sporting governing bodies for alleged restraint of trade offences (*Willander v Tobin* [1997] 1 Lloyd's Rep 195; *Edwards v BAF and IAAF* (*Daily Telegraph*, 24 June, 1997)). Each was unsuccessful for reasons outside the scope of this book, but two observations may be made:

1   Sport does not in itself qualify as an 'economic activity'.

2   Anomalies can arise, as in *Edwards v BAF and IAAF* (above) when the English shot putter, Paul Edwards, failed to persuade the court that a four-year ban by the IAAF was inconsistent with lesser periods ordered by German, Spanish and Russian courts.

The battle against those who use forbidden performance-enhancing techniques will no doubt continue. The detrimental side-effects of the use of steroids must be constantly stressed, in order that sportspeople who are tempted to use them will understand that a better performance is not the only effect of this practice.

At the time of writing, disturbing new evidence was emerging over the alleged systematic misuse of steriods and other proscribed drugs, organized by sports practitioners and coaches in the former East Germany (GDR). If the allegations bear scrutiny, it appears that doctors (and, indeed, State officials) were involved, not only in the illegal enhancement of sports performance by the use of drugs with known serious side effects, but also the wholesale and covert experimentation on the nation's pre-athletic youth in an attempt to establish links between specific compounds and future athletic performance. Indeed, while these pages are being prepared for publication a trial has begun in Berlin of two doctors and four coaches, charged with causing grievous bodily harm to minors by giving them steroids, with proven prospects if convicted of up to three years in jail (*Times*, 19 March, 1998).

When yet another sportsperson is tested positive, the public become resigned to the view that certain sports are not 'clean' and subsequently suspect that innocent participants may themselves be cheating. Undoubtedly, the real victims of this crime are the competitors who choose to compete using their own natural resources and refuse to compromise their integrity.

On that issue an argument has been formulated that any competitor who is downgraded, with consequential disadvantages to their financial sponsorship, who can prove loss would have a cause of action for negligence giving rise to damages. Dubin J's report concluded at p. 517:

> Cheating in sport, I fear, is partially a reflection of today's society. Drugs and the unprincipled pursuit of wealth and fame at any cost now threaten our very social fabric. It is little wonder the immorality has reached into sport as well. Of course, cheating as such is not a new phenomenon in Olympic competition, but the methods used to cheat have become more and more innovative and more pervasive. Moreover the use of drugs as the method of cheating has reached epidemic proportions.

If there is a solution, then what better remedy can be found than that proposed by Hubert Doggart OBE, President of the English Schools Cricket Association, an ex-Headmaster of King's School, Bruton, and nephew of the late James Doggart, FRCS, Ophthalmic Specialist, writing in Appendix I to *Sport and the Law* (Grayson, 1994, 2nd edn) under the title of *The Corinthian Ideal*:

> Three specific groups whose efforts could be harnessed to stop the rot and ensure the survival, relatively intact, of the Corinthian ideal.
>
> First, the doctors, whose Hippocratic oath can be construed as an upholding of the Corinthian ideal in medicine. Secondly, the lawyers, who once played without a thought that their services qua lawyers would be needed, but cannot now be sure. And, third, school teachers, whose raison d'être could be called 'the upholding of the Corinthian ideal in body, mind and soul'.

Finally, the concentration on drug abuse, with its health, ethical and moral implications, can divert attention from the concurrent problems of violence and cheating through violation of the rules of play. Indeed, there are many who consider that breaches of the rules by physical foul play has an even more damaging effect on sport than drug abuse because of its effect on youthful emulators.

Almost daily, and frequently weekly, referrals come the author's way from all parts of the UK to illustrate the increasing incidence of field violence. The following pages provide but a few examples.

## THE RULE OF LAW IN SPORT
**Applied to injury examples proved or alleged to have been caused by a breach of playing and/or national laws.** *A: Criminal*; *B: Civil* **(reproduced and updated from Grayson, Edward:** *Sport and the Law* **[2nd edn, 1994] Butterworths: by kind permission of the publisher)**

### A: Criminal

**1878**
*R v Bradshaw* (1878) 14 Cox CC 83 Leicester Assizes
*Facts*       Prosecution for unlawful soccer tackle: manslaughter charged.
*Decision*    Acquittal.
*Principle*   Deliberate and/or reckless tackle not proved to jury. Rider by jury to tighten up tackling rules.

**1882**
*R v Coney* (1882) 8 QBD 534 Berkshire Quarter Sessions
*Facts*       Bare-knuckle prize fight. Prosecution of spectators for aiding and abetting in such fight.
*Decision*    Conviction quashed for defective summing up.
*Principle*   Blow struck in prize fight clearly an assault, but playing with single sticks or wrestling does not involve an assault, nor does boxing with gloves in the ordinary way. Consent of illegal prize-fighters to interchange of blows no defence.

**1898**
*R v Moore* (1898) 14 TLR 229 Leicester Assizes
*Facts*       Prosecution for unlawful soccer tackle: murder.
*Decision*    Guilty. Manslaughter.
*Principle*   Deliberate and/or reckless tackle outside laws of game proved.

**1901**
*R v Roberts* (1901) *Daily Telegraph*, 29 June Central Criminal Court
*Facts*       Test case prosecution against National Sporting Club for illegality or legality of Queensberry rules boxing competition.
*Decision*    Acquittal.
*Principle*   Boxing within the rules as distinct from boxing until exhausted not unlawful.

**1969**

*R v Southby* (1969) 77 *Police Review* 110; 120 *NLJ* 413 Maidstone Assizes (transferred from Chelmsford)

*Facts*    Prosecution for murder after death from niggling blow in Essex amateur soccer match.

*Decision*    Guilty. Manslaughter.

*Principle*    Deliberate and/or reckless blow outside laws of game proved.

**1977***

*French Prosecutor v Palmie* (*Guardian*, 14 December, p. 19) Lyons, France

*Facts*    Prosecution of rugby international for field assault.

*Decision*    Conviction (reversed on appeal).

*Principle*    Deliberate and/or reckless foul play on field equals criminal conduct.

**1978**

*R v Billinghurst* [1978] Crim. Law R 553 Newport Crown Court

*Facts*    Prosecution for broken jaw in rugby tackle.

*Decision*    Conviction (not to be appealed).

*Principle*    As above – deliberate and/or reckless foul play on field equals criminal conduct.

**1980**

*R v Gingell* [1980] Crim. Law R 661 Croydon Crown Court; Court of Appeal

*Facts*    Prosecution for three fractures to face in rugby tackle: Guilty plea.

*Decision*    Immediate custodial sentence (six months). Confirmed in principle, reduced to two on appeal because first precedent (*quaere*: why only six: why not more?).

**1980**

*R v Doble* (unreported) Stafford Crown Court, 8–10 September, 1980 Wolverhampton Crown Court

*Facts*    Prosecution for gouging out eye in rugby tackle.

---

*This French case has no binding authority on the English courts. Because the prosecution was supported by the French Rugby Union against one of its international players later selected to play against England in the International Ruby Tournament, it is included to remind all aggressively-minded players and their friends in the Press Box, as well as all other national sporting bodies, of the potential and ultimate consequence of violent and unlawful conduct on sports fields.

*Decision*   Jury acquitted in spite of evidence.
*Principle*   Judge recommended victim to approach Criminal In-
              juries Compensation Board.


## 1982
Scottish Sheriff's Court (unreported)
*Facts*      Prosecution of two opposing rugby captains: prosecuted
             on advice of Procurator-Fiscal.
*Decision*   No evidence offered against one. Other pleaded guilty:
             suspended sentence.
*Principle*  Action at last: against punch-up on field (hitherto not
             pursued by abdication of prosecution responsibilities
             and also by victims for younger generations).


## 1985
FA Tribunal
*Facts*      Complaint by one professional footballer of assault by
             another within framework of bringing game into dis-
             repute under FA Rule 35(a) (unreported).
*Decision*   Not proven, but deposit returned to complainant on
             establishing *prima facie* case.
*Principle*  Action at last: recognition of existence of potential
             offence at professional level.


## 1985
Dursley, Gloucestershire, Magistrates' Court (unreported)
*Facts*      Private prosecution for broken leg in soccer tackle.
*Decision*   Guilty: £180 fine with costs.
*Principle*  Action at last: by victim on own initiative.


## 1985
Clacton, Essex Magistrates' Court (unreported)
*Facts*      Prosecution against women footballer for breaking
             opponent's jaw in women's 'friendly' soccer match.
*Decision*   Guilty: £250 compensation and costs.


## 1986
South Wales
*Facts*      Process initiated against Welsh International rugby
             player for alleged assault in club match.
*Decision*   Guilty plea to common assault.
*Principle*  First prosecution against international in UK.

## 1985–86
*R v Bishop* (1986) *Times*, 12 October Newport Crown Court; Court of Appeal

*Facts*      Concussion from punch in off-the-ball rugby union incident.

*Decision*  Guilty plea to common assault. Sentence: One month's custodial imprisonment reduced without reasons to one month's suspended imprisonment.

## 1986
*R v Johnson* [1986] 8 CAR (5) 343

*Facts*      Ear bitten after tackle in police rugby union match. Inflicting grievous bodily harm with intent contrary to s. 18 of the Offences against the Person Act 1861.

*Decision*  Convicted. Six months' custodial imprisonment. Confirmed on appeal.

## 1988
*R v Kamara* (1988) *Times*, 15 April Swindon Magistrates' Court

*Facts*      Broken jaw by professional soccer player in tunnel after match.

*Decision*  Guilty plea. Inflicting grievous bodily harm contrary to s. 20 of the Offences Against the Person Act, 1861.

## 1988
*R v Lloyd* (1988) *Times*, 13 September Bristol Crown Court

*Facts*      Broken cheekbone caused by amateur rugby player in club match kicking opponent on ground during course of play.

*Decision*  Conviction: grievous bodily harm. Eighteen months' imprisonment.

## 1988
*R v Birkin* (1988) *Enfield Gazette*, 7 April Wood Green Crown Court

*Facts*      Broken jaw by amateur soccer player in 'friendly' match.

*Decision*  Actual bodily harm.

## 1989
*R v Chapman* (CA transcripts) St Albans Crown Court; Court of Appeal

*Facts*      Concussion from kick on head to player on ground by soccer opponent.

*Decision*  Grievous bodily harm. Eighteen months' custodial sentence.

**1991**

Criminal Injuries Compensation Board (1991) NLJ 1725, Hals Laws MR 92/54

*Facts*       Eye gouged out from Rugby Union foul play in line-out
*Decision*   Criminal liability admitted though offender not identified. £15 000 interim compensation award.

**1994**

*RN v Russell* (1994) *Times*, 23 February RN Plymouth Court Martial

*Facts*       Broken nose from Rugby Union foul play.
*Decision*   Four months' detention. Reduced ranks.

**PARTICIPATION PROBLEMS: CIVIL DAMAGES
AWARDS FOR INJURIES
(adapted and extended from Grayson (1994))**

**B: Civil**

The following cases illustrate various compensation awards made for sports-related injuries.

**1927**

*Cleghorn v Oldham* (1927) 43 TLR 465

*Facts*        Golfer not in course of play swings club during demonstration and injures person standing by.
*Decision*    Player liable.
*Principle*   Not in course of play. Defence rejected of consent to negligent act not unfair or vicious in recreation. Negligent misconduct actionable in recreation as in any other activity.

**1949**

*Payne & Payne v Maple Leaf Gardens Ltd* (1949) 1 DLR 369 Canada

*Facts*        Ice hockey players stepped out of or broke off from hockey game to fight, injuring spectator with stick.
*Decision*    Players liable.
*Principle*   No consent to breach of rules.

**Pre-1962**

Unreported decision of Seller LJ on South Eastern Circuit (see [1963] 1 QB 43 at 55)

*Facts*     Golfer in four-ball hit into rough, losing the ball. Said: 'Out of it' and encouraged better players to proceed. Resumed after finding ball, causing injury as victim turned round at defendant's cry of 'Fore'.

*Decision*  Player liable.

*Principle* Conduct outside the game; unnecessary for it; showed complete disregard for safety of those he knew were in line of danger from being hit from an unskilled instead of lifted shot over their heads.

**1968**

*Lamond v Glasgow Corporation* (1968) SLT 291

*Facts*     Pedestrian walking along narrow public lane injured on head by golf ball.

*Decision*  Occupier liable for negligence.

*Principle* Although no previous history of any accident, 6000 shots a year played over fence should have created forecast of foreseeable happening.

**1981/2**

*Harrison v Vincent* [1982] RTR 8

*Facts*     Passenger in sidecar during motor cycle and sidecar combination race injured.

*Decision*  Motorcycle rider competitor and also race organizers liable.

*Principle* Rider and employers failed in duty to take care of condition of competing vehicle.

**1982**

*Bidwell v Parks* (unreported, except in newspapers) Lewes Crown Court, French J.

*Facts*     Golfer in tournament injured by ball hit from fellow competitor without warning.

*Decision*  Fellow competitor golfer liable.

*Principle* Dangerous for 24 handicap golfer to take shot which could have gone anywhere without warning.

**1983**

*Hewish v Smailes* (provided from court archives by H H Judge John A. Baker DL) Epsom County Court

*Facts*     Head-butt causing broken nose and black eyes to 38-year-old local player in local league match.

*Decision*    Civil assault (trespass to the person) damages claim: £400 general damages and £580 proved special damages and costs.

**1989**

*Vermont v Green* (provided by Mr Oliver Wise, Barrister) Basingstoke County Court

*Facts*    Kick during course of play to opponent causing two nights in hospital.

*Decision*    Civil assault (trespass to the person) damages claim: £400 general damages; but claim for aggravated damages refused.

*Principle*    Adjudicated to have been deliberate on spur of moment.

**1989**

*Thomas v Maguire and Queen's Park Rangers* [1989] *Daily Mirror*, 17 February High Court, London.

*Facts*    Damaged ligaments to professional footballer (Tottenham Hotspur).

*Decision*    Negligence claim based on illegal tackle. Agreed damages £1300 settled out of court.

**1990**

*May v Strong* (Halsbury's Laws MRE 92/62 All Eng AR (1991) p. 313) Teesside Crown Court

*Facts*    Broken leg – amateur soccer player.

*Decision*    £10 000 damages to 19-year-old semi-professional footballer (£6000 pain, suffering and loss of earnings: for compound fracture of tibia and fibula £4000, special damages for net loss earnings of nine months).

*Principle*    Serious foul play and violent conduct sent off field by referee equals recklessness – held by judge as assault.

**1994**

*O'Neill v Fashanu and Wimbledon Football Club* (1994) *Independent*, 14 October High Court, London.

*Facts*    Settlement of claim without admission of liability.

*Decision*    Negligence claims bases on alleged illegal tackle.

*Principle*    £70 000 agreed out-of-court settlement of claim without admission of liability after plaintiff's case and first defendant's disciplinary record admitted in evidence by Collins J.

**1994**

*R v Piff* (1994) *Guardian*, 2 February Court of Appeal Criminal Division

| | |
|---|---|
| *Facts* | Facial fractures admitted. Probation and compensation order. |
| *Decision* | Attorney General's reference to Court of Appeal custodial sentence substituted. Compensation Order cancelled. |

**1995**

*R v Ferguson* (1995) *Herald*, 25 May Scottish Sheriff's Court

| | |
|---|---|
| *Facts* | Head-butting professional football opponent. |
| *Decision* | Guilty after jury trial. Custodial prison sentence. |

**1996**

*R v Devereux* (1996) *Times*, 26 February Kingston-upon-Thames Crown Court

| | |
|---|---|
| *Facts* | Rugby player jaw-breaking assault. |
| *Decision* | Guilty after jury trial. Nine months' custodial sentence confined to appeal. |

**1996**

*McCord v Swansea City* High Court, London

| | |
|---|---|
| *Facts* | Professional football negligence claim against injuries, based on illegal tackle. |
| *Decision* | £250 000 damages award. |

**1996**

*Smolden v Whitworth and Nolan Under 19 Colts*

| | |
|---|---|
| *Facts* | Rugby injury. |
| *Decision* | Referee liable. |
| *Principle* | Failed to observe laws of the game for under 19 colts players. |

**1998**

*Watson and Bradford City v Gray and Huddersfield Town, Times*, 29 October Leeds High Court

| | |
|---|---|
| *Facts* | Professional football negligence award for mistimed tackle breaking opponent's leg. Claim for alleged interference and contractual relations rejected. |
| *Decision* | Agreed interim £50 000 damages. |

# Chapter 2

# WMA Guideline 1

**1 The physician who cares for sportsmen or athletes has an ethical responsibility to recognize the special physical and mental demands placed upon them by their performance in sports activities.**

This self-evident proclamation consistent with Dr Joseph Farber's WMA's 'working paper's' general *Code of Ethics for Sports Medicine*, and medical ethics generally, has built-in to it a cascade of differences which embrace the whole range of health and physical education from the cradle to the grave. It also creates a preamble or prelude to the remaining Guidelines for alerting sports medical practitioners in any category to the area or areas where different criteria and demands of treatment can exist. Thus, within the 113 different sporting activities identified by the Customs and Excise VAT rebate provisions, the 2nd edition of the USA *Sports Medicine for the Primary Care Physician* edited by Richard B. Birrer (1994, CRC Press) identifies in Appendix II p. 587 its four different types of sports categories specified herewith:

I   collision;

II   contact;

III   endurance;

IV   nonendurance/sedentary.

Accordingly, save for the trauma created by any violent impact beyond the normal sporting activity, the sports practitioner in any discipline should be ready to give treatment for injuries sustained in each of these different categories.

In an editorial footnote Birrer explained how the classification of sports into these categories:

> represents a summary of average performance levels. Many sports could be placed in alternative categories under special circumstances. For example, the use of light weights numerous times during weight-lifting would classify weightlifting as an endurance sport (i.e. circuit

weight training); while the practice of a soft martial arts style such as pakua would make it classified as an endurance sport.

In the following section, different sports are categorized according to the above scheme.

## TYPES OF SPORTS

### Category I – Collision
Boxing
Football (tackle)
Martial arts – 'full contact'

### Category II – Contact
Basketball
Baseball/softball
Wrestling
Soccer
Rugby
Lacrosse
Judo
Football – flag
Martial arts
Volleyball
Parachuting
Hockey
Cricket

### Category III – Endurance
Trampolining
Track and field events
Jogging/walking
Sledding/tobogganing/luge
Racquet sports
Skateboarding
Cycling
Surfing
Swimming
Skating (roller/ice)
Rowing
Diving – scuba
Skiing
Water polo
Gymnastics

Handball
Climbing/hiking/mountaineering/orienteering
Ultimate frisbee
Kayak
Dance
Cheerleading
Auto racing

**Category IV – Nonendurance/sedentary**
Golf
Bowling
Ballooning
Croquet
Gliding
Fishing
Flying
Yoga
Sailing
Diving
Shooting
Weightlifting
Horseshoe pitching
Caving
Camping
Billiards/snooker
Archery
Equestrian activities

Within each category, the practitioner must give due consideration to other factors concerning, for example, the *way* in which the
player participates in sport (i.e. whether as a professional or
amateur; whether individually or in a team; whether for significant
financial reward, etc) Such factors contribute to the participators
'sporting profile' and it is a full understanding of this which
practitioners need if their duty towards their patients is to be
properly discharged.

Amateur and professional participants' requirements must be
properly assessed. The immediate financial consequences in the
form of lost income resulting from inadequate sports medical
treatment and sporting injuries may be more dramatic at the
professional activity level; but employment losses may be no less
significant for the amateur participant.

Patients within a team or group structure can create a potential
conflict between the patient's requirements and the demands of a
team, club or other employer of a medical practitioner. The

practitioner's overriding duty at all times must be to the patient. Potentially, the position is analogous to the industrial, insurance, prison or service practitioner, since all operate within a two-dimensional obligation.

Illustrations of these differences are inexhaustible and will emerge at various stages during the subsequent WMA guidelines; but examples here suffice to demonstrate the different 'special physical and mental demands placed upon them by their performance in sports activities'.

It is also important for the practitioner to have an awareness and recognition within the different sports and their categories of:

1 the amateur–professional dichotomy;

2 gender differences/distinctions;

3 children;

4 youth;

5 adult;

6 veteran;

7 disabled; and

8 drug-related problems.

Each of those categories of classification will now be considered in turn.

## 1   *The amateur–professional dichotomy*

Boxing is a classic case. The limitation of organized amateur contests to three rounds with headguards contrasts with the professional contests for a longer duration without headguards, although each demands a medical licence for an established governing body.

## 2   *Gender differences/distinctions*

Physiological differences and distinctions within different sporting governing body criteria are self-evident, separate and apart from such further complexities as those emanating from, for example, gender reassignment surgery. The issues here were illustrated by the medical evidence which proved the conversion of Dr Richard Rasskind, a New York ophthalmic surgeon and skilled tennis player, to Dr Renee Richards (see *Richards v US Tennis Association and others* (1977) 400 NYS (2nd) 267). The position of the transsexual is further discussed by Mason and McCall-Smith (1994) at pp. 42ff.


3    *Children*

Clearly, sensitive and special attention is required to avoid assessment for treatment of children as if they were miniature adults. Thus, a special MOSA report in 1979 identifying the risk of serious injury in rugby football resulted in awareness of the need for insurance (a position also adopted by the RFU) and, ultimately, the celebrated case of *Van Oppen v Bedford School Trustees* [1989] 1 All ER 273. The school was exonerated, on the facts, from allegations of negligent coaching techniques and non-insurance. It was held that the school was not negligent in its coaching techniques and not liable for the injuries because they were the result of an accident, rather than the negligence of any party. Similarly, negligence for non-insurance was not found because there was no greater duty to insure on the school than there would be on the part of a parent. The case is discussed further in Grayson (1994) pp. 104, 108. After a period of silence and quiescence, MOSA in early 1997 re-appeared as an active voice in school sport. Furthermore, as the burn-out syndrome of Andrea Jaeger, Tracey Austin and Jennifer Capriati illustrates, the pressures at public level are self-evident. (See also Chapter 10, p. 119 concerning Guideline 13.)

Finally, a potential area for abuse in this category was illustrated by the evidence produced during the prosecution at Cardiff Crown Court and conviction of the former Olympic swimming coach Paul Hickson for having abused young swimmers (*Times* 25 September 1995). He was jailed for 17 years initially, reduced on appeal to 12.


4    *Youth*

Different stages and levels of physical and mental development demand awareness of potential mis-match in height and weight. This was illustrated by the damages award to the victim of the excessive enthusiasm demonstrated by a rugby playing schoolmaster in tackling a boy which resulted in a negligent liability judgment (*Affuto-Nartoy v Clark and ILEA* (1984) *Times*, 9 February). A further example is the award made during 1996 against a rugby union referee for allowing excessive scrum collapses in breach of the laws of the game, resulting in paralysis in the victim (*Smoldon v Whitworth and Nolan*, p. 57 *supra*).


## 5   *Adult*

Avoidable injuries created by breaches of the rules of play can create civil, criminal and Criminal Injuries Compensation Board compensation awards (see Chapter 1).


## 6   *Veterans*

Practitioners should favour encouragement rather than discouragement in accordance with current medical practice and developments, but within a structured programme. Such policy also reflects the movement towards the BMA concept of 'sport and exercise medicine'. Exercise for health individualized with risk factors in sport means competition associated with risk. (See further, Professor Archie Young *Medicine for Sport for Medicine* Lecture, 8 July, 1996, Institute of Sports Medicine, p. 14 *et seq*. Young and Susan Dinan, 'Fitness for Older People', *ABC of Sports Medicine*, 69–71: 1995; *Medical Care for the Elderly*: Hall, McLennan, Lye, 1993.)


## 7   *Disabled*

There should be recognition of the limited capacity of disabled participators and treatment should not be on the level of able-bodied participants (see *Morell v Owen*, discussed in All ER Annual Review 1992, p. 392 and *Times*, 14 December, 1993). In that case, liability was established against the particular governing body for disabled atheletes for their negligent organization of the events in question.


## 8   *Drug-related problems*

See also Chapter 6 and necessity of observing sporting governing body guidelines and regulations, balanced by necessity for *bona fide* medication and also breaches by governing bodies of regulations (e.g. *Modahl v British Athletic Federation* 1995: *New Law Journal* Vol. 145, 20 January).

These categories and citations are not intended to be exhaustive. Rather, they are illustrative of the illimitable range of activities which fall within the initial WMA guideline namely: 'The physician who cares for sportsmen or athletes has an ethical responsibility to recognize the special physical and mental demands placed upon them by their performance in sports activities'. Indeed, these categories can also be linked to Guideline 13, relating to regulatory action and to Macleod's additional 'Guideline 14',which obliges doctors to refer to the appropriate evidence of defective equipment, from surfaces to footwear and the need for protection such as gum-shields and goggles; and the reporting of deliberate foul play, together with imbalances in size and age groups of participants playing.

Chapter 3

# WMA Guideline 2

**2  When the sports participant is a child or an adolescent, the physician must give first consideration to the participant's growth and stage of development.**

**2.1  The physician must ensure that the child's stage of growth and development, as well as his or her general condition of health can absorb the rigours of the training and competition without jeopardizing the normal physical or mental development of the child or adolescent.**

**2.2  The physician must oppose any sports or athletic activity that is not appropriate to the child's stage of growth and development or general condition of health. The physician must act in the best interest of the health of the child or adolescent, without regard to any other interest or pressure from any other source.**

These criteria may seem self-evident and self-explanatory. Yet in the global, competitive village created by television, the demands of parental and coaching pressures can prove difficult to reconcile with the above guidelines. The premature burn-out syndrome is well publicized at public levels. American tennis superstars and central European gymnasts come readily to mind. Less visible are the countless aspiring competitors who may never achieve the ultimate goal of prestigious or financial success which their parents or coaches may wish for them. Nevertheless, the pressures on their health would have been no different from those imposed on their higher profile contemporaries. The abuses, potential and actual, which exist here are exhumed with harrowing and poignant details in Joan Regan's *Little Girls in Pretty Boxes*, sub-titled '*the making and breaking of elite gymnasts and figure skaters*' (1996).

Against that general background there are two separate sources comparable to Mason and McCall-Smith's classification of medical negligence categories which provide detailed particulars for illustrating the WMA guidelines on what amounts to child care within sport (Mason and McCall-Smith, 1994). One is from the BMJ *ABC of Sports Medicine* (1995); the other from Vivian Grisogono's *Children and Sport* (Grisogono, 1994).

## CLASSIFICATION

In the first classification source mentioned in the previous section, Professor Leslie Klenerman, under the section entitled 'Musculo-skeletal injuries in child athletes', concludes with five separate precautions for preventing overuse injury in children:

- Careful supervision by coaches and parents.
- Equipment checked regularly for fit and wear.
- Practice intensity and duration increased only gradually.
- Poor technique or posture recognized and corrected.
- Warm up and stretch exercises before and after sport.

In a chapter entitled 'Why do children get injured?' Grisogono (1994) tripled those five preventive overuse precautions into fifteen different reasons, summarized thus:

- Doing the wrong sport.
- Doing the wrong type or amount of sport for the stage of development.
- Using the wrong size of equipment.
- Too much sport.
- Lack of appropriate protective equipment.
- Inadequate skill training.
- Inappropriate fitness training.
- Insufficient preparation.
- Inadequate supervision.
- Poor discipline.
- Inappropriate size-match.
- Unsafe environment.
- Poor shoes.
- Playing when injured or not fully recovered from injury.
- Playing when over-tired or ill.

These causative factors for child injury serve as a warning for any sort of practitioner concerned with the medical welfare of children. Because medical evidence at any level arises by patient referral or general media profile, the legal illustrations of these practices and principles arise only when highlighted in court at a recognized extra-judicial tribunal, such as a GMC disciplinary hearing.

Three illustrations have already been cited under Guideline 1 in Chapter 2: *Affuto-Nartoy v Clark and ILEA* (1984) *Times*, 9 February identified the inappropriate size-match. MOSA rugby insurance recommendations, resulting in *Van Oppen v Bedford School* [1989] 1 All ER 273, emphasized a comprehensive survey. It directed attention to the role of the school doctor who may find himself affected by subsequent ethical guidelines analogous to the industrial, insurance, prison or services doctor in an employed capacity dealing with another doctor's patient (see Guidelines 7–9 below). The rugby union referee failed to understand and apply Rugby Union football's special laws for scrum collapses as modified on medical evidence for under-19 colt players (*Smolden*: pp. 22–23).

From the USA, a classic illustration of the inadequacies of school medical services resulted in a damages award of \$325 000 in 1958. The defendant school was held vicariously liable because the school doctor and coach were present when a high school football quarterback sustained a neck injury. The doctor in particular did not respond with sufficient alacrity to examine the victim or provide adequate immediate medical care for the (commonly enough sustained) neck injury which, in the particular case, resulted in permanent quadriplegia (*Welch v Dunsmuir Junior High School Dist* (1958) 326 P 2d 633).

The present writer was instructed to advise a visiting schoolboy rugby player seriously injured when he collided with the concrete base of the fence dividing the rugby player areas from an adjoining tennis court. The base was placed on the dead ball line beyond the rugby goal posts. No-one had pointed out to the school authorities the inherent danger in that position, and inevitably the claim was settled in the victim's favour.

More serious, was the conviction at Cardiff Crown Court and custodial sentence of seventeen years passed on a former Olympic swimming coach for abusing young swimmers, of which warning signs had been raised nine years earlier, without response from the appropriate sporting governing body (*R v Hickson* (1985) *Times*, 28 September). How far this disclosed an unseen and unknown depth of potential danger within the world of personal contact sports associated with young people is an issue which cannot be ignored.

Finally, indicative of the scope of the medical issues concerning children in sport were the near 40 special papers addressed at a two-day conference during July 1995 at the University of Bath Centre for Continuing Education, where a Sports Medicine for Doctors course has existed since 1992 (devised by Professor J. Ring).

Furthermore, during the time of the 1996 Atlanta Olympic Games, Tim Harding in the *Lancet*, Vol. 348: 10 August, 1996 at p. 400 drew attention to the recommendations of A. Franck and H. Olagnier from St Etienne, France in their *Medecine et Hygiene* (1996 : 54 : 1393–96):

> Most top-level athletes start their careers as adolescents. The problems associated with high level sport include exercise induced delay in growth, complex musculoskeletal injury; side effects of performance-enhancing drugs, and psychological damage. They readily become victims of parents' ambitions, the demands of trainers and totalitarian control of the federation of their sport. Training damages adolescents' social life, psychological development and physical health.

Accordingly, Franck and Olagnier believed that these abuses arose:

> because of the absence of free and informed consent and in the context of a pathological state of dependence on trainers and sports federations.

They therefore made six recommendations which, as Harding commented, 'may seem severe; but they reflect the author's concerns about serious and undescribed abuses':

1    Recognition that young adolescents are still children who are unable to consent fully to a training programme that will entail years of punishing and time-consuming exercise, which will inevitably distort their normal pyscho-social development.
2    Respect of professional ethical principles by doctors and psychologists involved in training programmes, in particular guarantees of professional independence and of medical confidentiality.
3    Legal protection for adolescent sports athletes that would be analogous to that existing for young actors, circus artists and musicians.
4    Adequate representation of parents through independent associations and full unbiased information available for all parties.
5    A control commission set up by the government [i.e. of any country] that is independent of sports federations [or, in the UK, Sports Councils the Central Council of Physical Recreation (CCPR) and the British Olympic Association (BOA)].
6    Creation of a multidisciplinary ethics committee attached to the International Olympics Committee.

Harding concluded:

> Much has been written about the distortion of sporting values under totalitarian communist regimes. Franck and Olagnier remind us that

totalitarian structures can exist in democratic societies, if they are supported by commercial interests and media pressures.

Indeed, Joan Regan's narrative reinforces this conclusion. Thus, there can never be any limit to the sports practitioner's duty to a child or adolescent within this particular WMA guideline 'to give his first consideration to the participant's growth stage of development'.

The following section gives examples of liability issues concerning children injured as a result of sporting activities.

## ISSUES CONCERNING CHILDREN INJURED AS A RESULT OF SPORTING ACTIVITIES
**(reproduced and updated from Grayson, Edward: *Sport and the Law* (2nd edn, 1994) Butterworths; by kind permission of the publisher)**

### 1932
*Langham v Governors of Wellingborough School and Fryer* (1932) 101 LKJB 513, 147 LT 91; 96 JP 236; 30 LGR 276

*Facts*     Unprecedented striking in a school playground of golf ball which hit eye of pupil inside a school building causing injury.
*Decision*     No liability.
*Principle*     School and staff exonerated from responsibility which could not have been prevented even by supervision.

### 1936
*Gibbs v Barking Corp* [1936] 1 All ER 115

*Facts*     Schoolboy during gymnastic training at school landed from a vaulting horse in 'a stumble', suffering personal injury.
*Decision*     Local authority liable.
*Principle*     Lack of promptitude by games master to prevent stumble when or after vaulting created lack of care causing accident and negligence.

### 1938
*Gillmore v London County Council* [1938] 4 All ER 331, 55 TLR 95, 159 LT 615

*Facts*     Fee-paying adult, participating in physical training class wearing rubber soles, slipped on fairly highly polished floor (suitable for dancing but not for physical exercise) which caused personal injury.
*Decision*     Organizing local authority council liable.

*Principle*    (1) Council failed in duty to provide a floor which was reasonably safe in circumstances creating danger beyond usual degree of playing a game.

(2) *Volenti non fit injuria* defence rejected because of consent to risk of this added danger beyond ordinary hazard lawfully practised.

**1939**

*Clark v Bethnal Green Corp* (1939) 55 TLR 519

*Facts*    Child at swimming bath let go suddenly of a springboard to which she had been clinging, thereby disrupting preparation to jump from it by another child who suffered injury.

*Decision*    No liability.

*Principle*    Action not capable of anticipation, irrespective of adequacy of supervision, for which evidence was equivocal and not definitive.

**1939**

*Barfoot v East Sussex CC* (unreported: *The Head's Legal Guide*: para. 3-111); Scott (1989) p. 221

*Facts*    School pupil injured when fielding at cricket, under supervision of teacher also acting a umpire. Evidence conflict between: (1) plaintiff pupil's claim of placed at 'silly mid-on' (facing batsman); (2) defendant's (per the master) of 'square leg' location (at right angles to wicket) and moving close to batsman of own accord.

*Decision*    Liability proved.

*Principle*    Umpire duties precluded exercise of sufficient supervisory care by the master in charge. They conflicted with need to prevent the boy being very considerably less than ten yards from wicket (as adjudged by court). This was a dangerous situation in the circumstances; and also in judgment of failure 'to exercise the care which the law required from a master in charge of pupils in these circumstances'.

N.B. Scott's industrious researches revealed that the trial judge, Humphreys J (Shrewsbury School XI) awarded damages for the plaintiff schoolboy after deciding 'with fear and trembling and with as much courage as I can assume', to disagree with the expert evidence testimony of the famous Sussex and England all-round player, Maurice Tate.

**1947**

*Ralph v LCC* (1947) 63 TLR 546, CA, 111 JP 548

*Facts* School game of 'touch' played in room with insufficient space and one participant placed hand unwittingly through glass partition causing injury.

*Decision* Liability proved.

*Principle* Reasonable and prudent father would have contemplated possibility of such an accident.

**1968**

*Beaumont v Surrey CC* (1968) 66 LGR 580, 112 SJ 704

*Facts* Horseplay during school break caused foreseeable injury of eye from discarded elastic rope because of breakdown in usually adequate school supervision.

*Decision* Liability proved.

*Principle* (1) Reasonable prudent parent principle (above) not applied to headmaster of school with 900 pupils.

(2) Duty breached, to take all reasonable and proper steps to prevent injury between pupils, bearing in mind known propensities of boys or girls between ages 11 and 18.

**1981**

*Moore v Hampshire CC* (1981) 80 LGR 481 C

*Facts* 12-year-old pupil with dislocated hip and unfit for physical training of which teacher advised. Wrongful persuasion that permission authorized and disability caused awkward movement resulting in injury.

*Decision* Liability proved.

*Principle* Double failure: (1) to observe awkward movements; (2) to supervise properly within special category as disabled child.

**1981**

*Tracey Moore v Redditch and Bromsgrove Gymnast Club* (unreported: but recorded to emphasize the value of insurance for victim and insured)

*Facts* 18-year-old gymnast injured when using trampoline facilities in gymnasium during period of supervision at gymnasium club.

*Decision* Out of court settlement.

*Principle* No admission of liability on negligence allegation. Claim £350 000. Insurance policy ceiling at £250 000. Settlement £250 000, with denial on liability that supervision inadequate.

**1984**

*Affuto-Nartoy v Clarke and ILEA* (1984) *Times*, 9 February

*Facts*      15-year-old schoolboy injured during school rugby game by high tackle from schoolmaster during instructional period, without any unfair play issue.

*Decision*  Liability proved.

*Principle*  Teacher momentarily forgot playing with young schoolboys of lesser and smaller physique than himself.

**1985**

*Condon v Basi* (1985) 2 All ER 453

*Facts*      Soccer player injured by foul play in club match sued for wrongful assault and negligence in claim for broken leg.

*Decision*  Liability proved.

*Principle*  Negligence upheld in Court of Appeal because of duty owed by one competitor to another to play according to the rules was breached on this occasion by violent foul play.

**1988**

*Van Oppen v Clerk to the Bedford Charity Trustees* [1989] 1 All ER 273; affirmed [1989] 3 All ER 389, CA

*Facts*      Schoolboy injured by rugby tackle but not insured.

*Decision*  Negligence not proved and alleged failure to insure rejected.

*Principle*  Evidence of no negligence. No duty to insure equivalent to non-parental duty to insure.

**1991**

*Gannon v Rotherham MBC Halsbury's Monthly Review* July 1991 91/1717

*Facts*      Schoolboy recovered damages against schoolteacher and governing body for broken neck in swimming bath injury.

*Decision*  Liability proved.

*Principle*  Inadequate supervision and guidance.

**1993**

*Morrell v Owen* (1993) *Times*, 14 December

*Facts*      Disabled wheelchair athlete injured by unsafe discus thrower.

*Decision*  Negligence proved.

*Principle*  Higher duty of care owned to athletes under disability than to able-bodied participants.

**1996**

*Smolden v Whitworth and Nolan* (1996) *Times*, 18 December, CA

*Facts*       Under-19 Rugby Colts player paralysed by collapsed scrum in breach of rules of the game.

*Decision*    Negligence proved

*Principles*   Breach of duty of care through ignorance of rules of game.

**1998**

*Williams v Rotherham LEA* (1998) *Times*, 6 August

*Facts*       Pupil forced to join PE lesson notwithstanding injured ankle.

*Decision*    Negligence proved.

*Principle*    Known aggravation of pre-existing injurous condition exacerbated physically injured ankle.

**1998**

*R v David Calton* (1998) *Yorkshire Post*, 29 September

*Facts*       Broken jaw suffered in rugby match between two leading Yorkshire private schools.

*Decision*    Crown Court Prosecution conviction. Sentence: 12 months Young Offenders Institution.

*Principle*    Law of land does not stop touchline, even for young offenders.

Chapter 4

# WMA Guideline 3

**3    When the sports participant is a professional sportsman or athlete and derives livelihood from that activity, the physician should pay due regard to the occupational medical aspects involved.**

Recently, Frank Bruno has announced his retirement from professional boxing on the considered advice of ophthalmic medical practitioners. Some years earlier, the former England rugby captain, Bill Beaumont, was advised to retire upon well publicized neurological advice because of a neck injury sustained when playing his particular game, albeit as an amateur outside a full-time business career; and Gordon Taylor, the chief executive of the Professional Footballers' Association (PFA) had announced on more than one occasion how thirty or forty professional footballers each year are forced to retire because of injuries suffered during their respective careers.

The implications of non-diagnosis of a latent defect seem obvious enough today. This position has evolved during the career of the present writer. When Derek King (previously of Tottenham Hotspur) was signed by Swansea City at the start of the 1956–57 football season, surprising as it seems today, he underwent no medical examination.

The Swansea club's history, 1912–1982, explains the events which followed:

> [King] played only five games at the Vetch Field before being forced to give up the game as a result of a knee defect ... the Swans claimed that King was unfit when he arrived, while the vendors held the opposite view. Unhappily for the Vetch men the contract was valid.

The contractual terms were not identified, but the absence of any medical examination by the purchasing club would be unheard of today. The Bolam test directs that a doctor 'is not negligent ... merely because there is a body of opinion who would take a contrary view' to his or her own. If a club doctor were to misdiagnose an ascertainable medical flaw when examining a player

74

before a transfer, and if within a reasonable time afterwards the player showed such a medical flaw, the doctor personally, and any employer club vicariously, could be at a substantial risk for any authentic loss suffered by the purchasing club, through loss of services or devaluation of the purchased player. A relatively recent example was the case of Paul Ince, where a £2 million transfer from West Ham United to Manchester United was frustrated by an apparent discovery of a pelvic injury upon a medical inspection. (Ince was eventually transferred after thorough medical investigations.)

Similarly, in 1977, Queen's Park Rangers failed to satisfy Laughton Scott J in the High Court that Sheffield Wednesday misled them into paying £55 000 for Vic Mobley, who had represented England at under-23 level, on the basis that his osteoarthritic knee condition had not been disclosed at the time of the transfer transaction. After a twenty-day trial, and a reserved judgment, which covered extensive medical evidence, the court concluded that Mobley disclosed no osteoarthritic symptoms at the time of the transfer. No appeal against the decision was lodged.

The equestrian sports of the National Hunt and steeplechasing have developed (through the Jockeys' Association) a dialogue with the Jockey Club and its successive medical officers in order to direct attention to the amelioration of injuries at race track facilities, barrier rails and in respect of every aspect of safety circumstances from helmets to course surfaces.

The British Boxing Board of Control (BBBC) and Amateur Boxing Association (ABA) regulate their respective jurisdictions and licensed boxers under their control with strict medical inspections and safeguards. Nevertheless, pending litigation from Michael Watson, who was grievously injured when boxing at the Tottenham Hotspur stadium, will disclose whether and, if so, to what extent there had been a failure of arrangements to transport him with sufficient speed and care to hospital for urgent neurosurgery. Efficient co-ordination and response to a complaint are inevitably as crucial in the area of sporting injuries as the treatment itself; and the vicarious liability decision of the Canadian courts against the Vancouver Hockey Club (*Robitaille v Vancouver Hockey Club Ltd*) illustrates graphically the failure to pay due regard to the 'occupational medical aspects involved'.

Furthermore, it is at least arguable that, clinically, no difference exists between the sports physician's regard to the 'occupational medical aspects involved' for an amateur participant whose sporting or sports-related injury can be as equally disastrous, as for the professional sports participant. Disablement to an injured accountant, dentist or doctor, lawyer or school teacher can be as relatively financially injurious as it can be for a professional athlete. Two illustrations from different dimensions illustrate the significance of the 'occupational medical aspects involved'. Dr J. C. Betts as Vice President of the British Sub Aqua Club contributed 'Scuba-diving and its medical problems: the role of the doctor' in *Medicine, Sport and the Law*, Blackwell Scientific Publications, 1990, pp. 295–6:

While the BSAC has been the subject of litigation on several occasions, these have usually involved indefensible diving procedures, usually novice divers taken into conditions totally unsuitable for them. There has only been one case of note involving the BSAC in which the medical aspects predominated. In many ways, this exemplifies the problems which may befall the unprepared casualty officer. An insulin-dependent diabetic business executive joined the BSAC at a time when, subject to certain safeguards, diabetics were still accepted as divers. While still an inexperienced diver, he went on a boat to dive to a depth of 30 m. Before diving he explained to his companions that he was a diabetic and that, if he became unconscious, he should be given sugar. He was accompanied on his dive by two very experienced members, who said that his maximum bottom time was not exceeded. On surfacing his legs became weak as he swam back to the boat and he had to be assisted on board where, shortly afterwards, he became unconscious. As instructed, he was given sugar and partly regained consciousness. It took some time to get him ashore, where he was taken to the local casualty department. Unfortunately his apparent response to sugar was misinterpreted as evidence of hypoglycaemia and he was given further quantities of glucose. It was not until several hours later that a blood glucose was taken and was found to be above 30 mmol/l. He was sent to the local recompression chamber, where he was found to be paraplegic. Unfortunately, management of a hyperglycaemic diabetic in recompression proved extremely difficult and there was no response to treatment. He emerged after three days almost tetraplegic, with only a little power in one hand. Eventually he committed suicide and his widow sued the BSAC, its officers, the diving officer and the buddy diver, the casualty officer and the area health authority.

The history of rapid onset of symptoms after a normally safe dive would suggest that he sustained an air embolism and the case was fought on this basis, although the subsequent post-mortem showed the changes of decompression sickness in the spinal cord. It is conceivable that this resulted later from his recompression treatment, compromised as it was by his gross hyperglycaemia.

Interestingly enough, no criticism was made in court of the original decision to accept him as a diabetic diver. Very substantial damages were awarded against the area health authority and casualty officer while the BSAC and its members were exonerated.

Subsequently the Medical Committee of the BSAC, when reviewing the case, felt that it had identified a hitherto unforeseen problem, namely the extreme difficulty of making a diagnosis in an unconscious diabetic diver at sea and advised the club that in the light of this case it would be indefensible to allow diabetics to continue as diving members of the club.

Martin J. Greenberg, Director of the National Sports Law Institute at Marquette University Law School, Wisconsin, USA, and a practising lawyer, was good enough to provide me with details of an American college football fatality suffered by Hank Gathers who was 'the epitome of the American dream'. The 23-year-old basketball superstar collapsed during a game on 4 March, 1990, and died one hour and forty-one minutes later. The cause of death was disputed between either myocarditis or hypertrophic cardiomyopathy. Three months earlier, on 9 December, 1989, Gathers had fainted during a basketball game against the University of California at Santa Barbara. He was diagnosed as having an irregular heartbeat condition, cardiac arrhythmia (athlete's heart). In due course, several of the doctors treating Gathers were accused of fraudulent concealment and conspiracy by virtue of their failure to disclose to Gathers the true nature and extent of his heart condition. Two consolidated suits involving twenty-nine attorneys and ten law firms were involved in litigation on behalf of his family. Loyola Marymount University, as the employer of the coach, athletic trainer and some doctors, were alleged to be vicariously liable if their alleged inadequate treatments were found to be within the scope of their employment responsibilities and ultimately proved to be negligent. (*Lucille Gathers, et al v Loyola Marymount, et al, Martin M Krimsky, Administrator for Estate of Eric Wilson Gathers, Jr, and Michael Horsey, Guardian of the Estate of Aaron Kevin Crump v Loyola Marymount University, et al,* Superior Court of the State of California, County of Los Angeles, Case No. C-759027.)

The Gathers case sent shock waves throughout the USA sports medical and general sporting college scene. As Greenberg recorded in the manuscript copy which he sent to me:

There is no question that Gathers has caused a fear among athletic personnel to permit time bomb athletes – athletes with potentially life-threatening medical conditions to compete. Here are a few guidelines and suggestions that should be followed. High school and university athlete programs should conduct pre-season physical examinations. However, a general medical examination may not provide sufficient information. It is recommended that an orthopaedic screening be completed by either an orthopaedic surgeon, certified athletic trainer or physical therapist. A typical orthopaedic examination would cover such areas as cardiovascular endurance, reflexes, muscular strength, flexibility, balance as well as joint and gait evaluations. Once a life threatening medical condition is detected, only outside medical experts who are treating the afflicted athlete can decide when the athlete may return to athletic competition. Athletic personnel can inquire about the medical condition of their athletes, however, they should not be involved in the medical decision of when an athlete can safely return to competition. If an athlete is diagnosed to be medically unfit to play, the university should legally be able to prevent the athlete from competing based upon its established safety standards and an appeal procedure based on due process where the athlete can challenge within the system the athletic personnel decision. If an athlete is determined to be medically fit to play based on a previously determined life threatening condition, a liability waiver should be executed, but drafted specifically for the subject medical problem at issue with full informed consent disclosures. And, finally, a word to all, it is better to err on the side of caution.

*Also from the USA*

A further final word also from the USA surfaced while these pages were in preparation in the form of a special section within a special edition of the valuable *Clinics in Sports Medicine* series related to *Neurological Athletic Head and Neck Injuries* edited by the Chief of Neurosurgery Service and Director of the Service of Sports Medicine at Emerson Hospital, Concord, Massachusetts, Robert C. Cantu. A chapter headed 'Medico-legal Aspects of Athletic Cervical Spine Injury' by a practising attoney Philip M. Davis, identified a range of litigation damages awards from a survey of football (American), diving, gymnastic, trampoline, waterskiing and snow skiing injuries, and concluded at p. 154:

> As a trial attorney, I have handled in excess of 200 catastrophic neck injuries resulting from football, baseball, gymnastics, wrestling and skiing. There will always be the risk of catastrophic injuries in sports. The very nature of many activities puts the participant at risk, however remote, of a paralysing neck injury. Because the risk is inherent in sports, it is crucial that everyone connected with the participant make their best effort to adequately warn the participant of the risks involved with the sport and offer proper instructions, warnings, coaching, and training techniques. Manufacturers of sporting goods equipment must place adequate warnings on all sporting goods they manufacture. Coaches should be educated in proper techniques, and they must pass their knowledge on to the participants. The reduction of cervical injury and the resulting litigation is the ultimate goal, which as the example of football rule changes and improved coaching techniques demonstrate can occur, and hopefully

at some point in the future may be substantially preventable in all sports.

On the basis that WMA Guideline 3 declares:

> When the sports participant is a professional sportsman or athlete and derives livelihood from that activity, the physician should pay due regard to the occupational medical aspects involved

the litigation examples of different participatory sports-related activity place the sports physician in a special relationship with the actual sport and patient under his or her care for the overriding philosophy of sports medicine to prevent as well as rehabilitate injury.

The final stages of preparation for this text re-affirmed the injury occupational consequences even to amateur, additionally to professional, participants. A *British Journal of Sports Medicine* case report in December 1998 (vol. 32, pp. 344–5) recorded in relation to a scuba diving shoulder injury how 'amateur scuba divers are considered to be at low risk because their dives are usually short and shallow'. It produced a commentary:

> Scuba diving is an increasingly popular sport worldwide. Most people who participate do so without any ill effects. However, the medical risks of an environment that imposes unique physical, physiological and psychological stresses on the body should not be forgotten.... The recent call by the Health and Safety Executive for proposals for research into the long-term health effects of diving is a welcome step in this direction, especially as some in the scuba diving community are using helium gas mixtures in an effort to reach even greater depths.

A brief case report of *Bacon v White (t/a Puffin Air)* (1998) in the *New Law Digest*, 14 June, 1998, recorded a 50 per cent liability against the organizers of a scuba diving event arising out of the death of a novice scuba diver. He had inaccurately completed a medical questionnaire prior to a diving course and had also, contrary to instruction, become separated from the rest of the group during a dive. Liability was established on the duty of care owed by instructors to novices.

Finally, consistent with the global significance of sports medicine and its impact internationally on all ages and occupations, the International Labour Office from Geneva in mid-1998 published the 4th edition of its mammoth four-volume *Encyclopaedia of Occupational Health and Safety*. The Preface began:

> It is a sobering thought that the prefaces to preceding (1930, 1972, 1983) editions of this *Encyclopaedia* are still timely: occupational

illnesses and injuries remain an unnecessary blight on the human landscape.

Volume 3 illustrates and describes four pages under the heading *Professional Sports* with the warning how 'Precautions, condition and safety equipment, when used properly will minimize sports injuries' [Part XVII, *Services and Trade*: 96. *Entertainment and the Arts*: pp. 96, 46–49].

Chapter 5

# WMA Guideline 4

**4 The physician should oppose the use of any method which is not in accordance with professional ethics, or which might be harmful to the sportsman or athlete using it, especially:**

**4.1 Procedures which artificially modify blood constituent or biochemistry.**

**4.2 The use of drugs or other substances whatever their nature and route of administration, including central-nervous-system stimulants or depressants and procedures which artificially modify reflexes.**

**4.3 Induced alterations of will or general mental outlook.**

**4.4 Procedures to mask pain or other protective symptoms if used to enable the sportsman or athlete to take part in events when lesions or signs are present which make his participation inadvisable.**

**4.5 Measures which artificially change features appropriate to age and sex.**

**4.6 Training and taking part in events when to do so would not be compatible with preservation of the individual's fitness, health or safety.**

**4.7 Measures aimed at unnatural increase or maintenance of performance during competition. Doping to improve an athlete's performance is unethical.**

Any medical or paramedical practitioner practising without an awareness of the daily conflicts between regulatory bodies in sport and society generally, and attempted evasions of prohibited substance controls, within and outside sport, exists on a different planet from the real world of today. The battle lines were further blurred than they had been before when the President of the International Olympic Committee, Juan Antonio Samaranch, exploded his bombshell already cited in the Preamble, here, ironically on the eve of the 50th anniversary of the opening of the first post-Second World War Olympic Games in London:

> Substances that do not damage a sportsman's health should not be banned.

One of Britain's leading and most respected international sports-writers, Ian Wooldridge, wrote in London's *Daily Mail* on that anniversary, 29 July, 1998 'He betrayed the youth of the world'.

The blurring was further evidence of the ambiguities which cloud the world of unthinking sporting administration, devoid of leadership apart from sports medical practitioners, illustrated at a United Kingdom Sports Council Seminar on 30 October, 1996 under the banner of 'Tackling Ethical Issues in Drugs and Sport'. Dr Malcolm Brown, Medical Adviser to the near bankrupt British Athletic Federation at the date of writing in receivership, explained:

> ... under the IAAF regulations as opposed to the IOC regulations and this is where problems sometime begin, there's no restriction on the use of inhaled cortico-steroids and rightly so. Oral cortico-steroids are not allowed and the mechanism by which you might have been able to persuade the IOCC to give exceptional permission, are not well publicised.

This, of course reflects the domestic dimension explained from West Sussex, England, cited at p. 41 (*supra*) in Chapter 1, of the need for general practitioners to be better informed of current and updated guidelines. Thus, if ever an example is required of what has now become a cliché, namely, that sport reflects society, the drug scenario mirrors it.

It should be noted that, in addition to the above ethical guidelines, some measures under certain national jurisdictions can also be unlawful. Thus, the UK Home Office, after an eight year gestation period outlawed anabolic steroids in 1995 in accordance with recommendations made in 1987. These are the most commonly known, but are far from being the only form of 'method which is not in accordance with professional ethics, or which might be harmful to the sportsman or athlete using it'. The use of drugs transcends the sports medicine and veterinary worlds, and is reflective of all social issues and attitudes. Whilst there are those in sports management who advocate the controlled use of performance enhancing drugs, the vast majority of sports medical practitioners are firmly against such a development. It demands attention and action at every level where medicine, sport and the law merge. Doctors, patients, parents, schools, club coaches, and governing bodies must all address the issues raised and the implications for modern sport.

Doctors in sport must be aware of the regulations which affect the administration of drugs in different sporting jurisdictions. Parents and schools, all acting *in loco parentis*, have duties to protect their infant charges. Club coaches and governing bodies owe a duty to their respective sports and those who participate in them to create practical regulations which are effective against the misuse of drugs but which do not preclude *bona fide* medical treatment when appropriate for general health circumstances.

Historically, the precedents exist for what is now a sophisticated battle between the scientific protection of those in participation, and those who would seek to take advantage of it by unfair methods.

Thus, the Canadian Government's *Commission of Inquiry in the Use of Drugs and Banned Substances Intended to Increase Athletic Performance* (1990) explained in its opening pages:

> The literature on doping in sport contains many historical references.
> For example, Melvin Williams, in *Drugs and Athletic Performance*,
> has written:
>> Ancient Greeks ate sesame seeds, the legendary Berserkers in
>> Norwegian mythology used bufotein, while the Andean Indians
>> and Australian Aborigines chewed, respectively, coca leaves and
>> the pituri plant for stimulating and antifatiguing effects. Catton, in
>> his classic Civil War account, indicated the Army of the Potomac
>> maintained its energy due to the tremendous amount of coffee the
>> soldiers consumed. From the early part of this century, boxers,
>> marathon runners, European cyclists, baseball and soccer players,
>> Olympic contestants and other athletes have used numerous
>> pharmaceutical agents as ergogenic aids. As an example, Tatarelli
>> experimented with a compound called Nike, consisting of vitamin
>> C, glucose, potassium acid tartrate, kola, and phosphorilamine, in a
>> study concerning the pharmaco-biological potentiation of the
>> athlete. However, it is only in recent years that drug use in athletics
>> has received considerable attention, probably because of the
>> national and international drug problem as a whole. There is no
>> doubt of course that drugs can and do enhance performance either
>> by creating a physical and advantageous edge to it or believing in a
>> psychological self belief advance.

Similarly, Michael J. Asken, in *Dying to Win* wrote of historical drug use:

> The ancient Greek physician Galen reported that athletes of the third
> century BC used stimulants. Herbs and mushrooms are reported to
> have been used to enhance performance by the Greek Olympians.
> Aztec athletes used a cactus-based stimulant resembling strychnine. In
> the mid and late nineteenth century, boxers used a brandy and cocaine
> mixture as well as strychnine tablets. Other coca leaf preparations
> were used in the late nineteenth century. Vin Mariani, a mixture of
> wine and coca leaf abstract, known as 'wine for athletes' was used by
> French cyclists. In 1904, marathoner Thomas Hicks competed
> successfully in the Olympics. It took four physicians to revive him

·after his success, however, because he had taken brandy and strychnine. In the 1930s, powdered gelatine mixed in orange juice was believed to be a performance enhancer. Athletes have also used sugar cubes dipped in ether. Sprinters have tried using nitro-glycerine to dilate the arteries of their hearts to improve performance. Ludwig Prokop, professor of sports medicine and director of the Austrian Institute of Sports Medicine in Vienna, reported that his first encounter with substance abuse was in athletes at the Oslo Winter Olympic Games in 1952. There he found broken ampoules and injection syringes in the locker room of speed skaters. He also reported seeing a classical case of strychnine cramp on the stage of the 1964 Weight Lifting World Championship. He writes of seeing the same evidence of drug abuse again in speed skaters at the 1964 Olympic Games in Innsbruck.

Neal Wilkinson commented on the 1956 summer games that:

> This craze for pills was most shocking at the recent Olympic Games. In Olympic village, the athletes' rooms looked like small drug stores. Vials, bottles and pill boxes lined the shelves.

The following list, by no means complete, includes some of the more conspicuous events in the modern history of doping in sport throughout the world.

1865   Swimmers in Amsterdam become the first documented modern case of doping. From this date into the early 1900s, swimmers, cyclists, and marathon runners are discovered using drugs, primarily stimulants.

1952   Winter Olympics in Oslo: anecdotes circulate about doping of speed skaters (see above).

1956   Summer Olympics in Melbourne: anecdotes about doping of cyclists.

1960   Summer Olympics in Rome: Danish cyclist Knut Jensen dies during competition after having ingested amphetamines and nicotinyl tartrate. The Council of Europe tables a resolution against the use of doping substances in sport.

1964   Summer Olympics in Tokyo: rumours of widespread drug use.

1965   Belgium and France enact antidoping legislation.

1966   Ireland passes antidoping regulations.

1967   The IOC Medical Commission is established. The Council of Europe passes a resolution on drug abuse in sport.

1968 The first IOC testing for stimulants and narcotics takes place at the Olympics in Grenoble and Mexico. One athlete disqualified for using alcohol.

1969 The Swiss Sports Association establishes domestic rules and regulations against doping.

1971 Italy and Turkey enact national antidoping legislation.

1972 The IAAF Medical Committee is formed. Winter Olympics in Sapporo: one athlete is disqualified for taking ephedrine. Summer Olympics in Munich: first large-scale analysis of urine samples at a major games (2079 samples). Seven athletes disqualified (see p. 88).

1973 The Council of Europe tables a definition of doping.

1974 IAAF and IOC medical commissions ban anabolic steroids use.

1975 Pan American Games in Mexico City: the first Canadian tests positive.

1976 Greece enacts national antidoping legislation.

Winter Olympics at Innsbruck: two athletes are disqualified.

Summer Olympics at Montreal: anabolic steroids tests are for the first time taken at an Olympic Games (only fifteen per cent of specimens are tested for anabolic steroids). Eleven athletes are disqualified, eight for anabolic steroids.

1977 The Swedish Sports Federation forms a doping control subcommission.

The Norwegian Confederation of Sports adopts a resolution on doping control.

West Germany sets out basic principles to fight against doping.

1978 The Danish Sports Federation establishes domestic rules and regulations against doping.

Sports Medicine Council of Canada is established.

1978 Willie Johnston, a Scottish International soccer player is expelled from the 1978 World Cup competition in Argentine by FIFA. He had been prescribed Reactavan tablets by his club doctor for an asthma condition. He was unaware that they contained Fencamsamin, a drug prohibited by FIFA regulations. When asked by the Scottish FA doctor whether or not he had taken a banned substance, his answer was in the negative. As his team manager, Ally McLeod, later explained in his own record of that competition 'Willie thought that they were no more harmful than Smarties'.

1979    Portugal enacts national antidoping legislation.

Deutscher Sportbund and Norwegian Sports Confederation establish domestic rules and regulations against doping.

1980    Winter Olympics at Lake Placid, Summer Olympics at Moscow: no disqualifications.

1981    Pacific Conference Games: the first Canadian is disqualified for use of anabolic steroids. The Swedish doping submission initiates out-of-competition testing.

1982    The Finnish Sports Federation establishes domestic rules and regulations against doping. The IOC introduces the first qualitative tests, for testosterone and caffeine.

1983    Pan American Games in Caracas, Venezuela: many athletes leave the games before competing to avoid tests; nineteen athletes are disqualified, including two Canadians.

1984    The Europe Anti-Doping Charter of the Council of Europe's committee of sports ministers is accepted. Summer Olympics at Los Angeles: twelve athletes are disqualified for doping; after the games, members of the medal-winning US cycling team admit blood doping. The English courts are required to remedy a reach of natural justice concerning a participant who had not been allowed to present his side of the case. Ron Angus, an international judo athlete was banned by the British Judo Association for use of the banned substance pseudo-ephedrine. He had not been given the opportunity to explain to the adjudicating tribunal how his prescription from a Canadian doctor (who treated him because of a dual Canadian-British nationality) was for a *bona fide* asthmatic condition; and his life ban is set aside in the High Court in the UK.

1985    Austria sets guidelines for fighting drug abuse in sport. Cyprus introduces drug testing.

1986    Canada's proposals for a world antidoping movement are endorsed at the European Sports Ministers Conference of the Council of Europe.

1987    The Socialist Nations Sports Ministers release a unified statement against doping.

US law enforcement agencies focus on the illegal market in anabolistic steroids and indict thirty-four people, including British Olympic medallist David Jenkins, in connection with importing and counterfeiting drugs.

The first IAF World Symposium on Doping in Sports is held in Florence, Italy.

1988 Canada hosts the First Permanent World Conference on Antidoping in Sport.

Ben Johnson's expulsion from the 1988 Olympic Games in Seoul occurs for his having taken a banned substance Stanazol. It results in a Canadian Government Commission of Inquiry, and ultimately disciplinary action for Johnson, his coach Francis and doctor, Astaphan.

Sandra Gasser, a Swiss athlete, banned by the IAAF from competition for having taken anabolic steroids, fails in the English High Court to reverse it.

1992 Katrin Krabbe, a German sprinter, successfully challenges the German Athletic Federation's expulsion provisions, in the German courts.

Harry Reynolds, challenges an IAAF banning decision, initially successfully but ultimately unsuccessfully in the American courts.

1995 Diane Modahl, an English sprinter, disqualified from the 1994 Commonwealth Games in Vancouver, successfully appeals to an administrative tribunal established by the British Athletic Federation, against an early banning decision because of the levels of testosterone found in a urine sample. The formal basis for her successful evidence was that the samples had become degraded owing to their having been stored in unrefrigerated conditions. An arguable basis which had been advocated but apparently ignored during each of two tribunal appearances was the absence of the conventional and regularly activated chain of custody. Before or shortly after these pages appear, a settlement of her appeal to the House of Lords or a judgment from it may well have been heard.

1998 A Canadian snowboarder is banned by the IOC for using marijuana, but because the substance is not listed as banned, the decision is countermanded. The Fédération Internationale de Natation Amateur (FINA) leaves sanction to Chinese authorities after banned drugs are found in the possession of

Chinese swimming team members by customs officials at Perth.

1998   World Medical Association, Ottawa Congress, debates drugs in sport (see Preface, pp. xiii–xiv).

1999   International Olympic Committee Conference is planned for February 1999.

1972 was the landmark year for drugs/doping in sport. In the *Dictionary of Medical Ethics* (2nd edn, 1981) and in the context of the IOC's Medical Commission, Professor Arnold H. Beckett, wrote under '*Sport: The Problems of Drugs In*' at p. 41:

... the following list of banned *classes* of doping agents was approved for the 1972 Olympic Games:
a) psychomotor stimulant drugs e.g. amphetamine etc.
b) sympathomimetic amines e.g. ephedrine etc.
c) miscellaneous central nervous system stimulants e.g. nikethamide, strychnine etc.
d) narcotic analgesics e.g. morphine etc.

In 1975, anabolic steroids were added to the classes. In all classes, the words 'and related compounds' were included after a variety of examples of each class. This is essential because otherwise compounds not intended as drugs but with the desired pharmacological effect would be used to circumvent the control based upon a comprehensive list of drugs.

The sympathomimetic amine class represents a special problem because of the use of some of the compounds of this class to treat colds and allergies. If, however, ephedrine were allowed as medication, in some sports a large dose would be used immediately to produce a stimulant effect. The policy is now to allow certain *specified* compounds to treat these problems so long as notification is made by a physician of their proposed use in a specified competitor.

Local anaesthetics are sometimes misused in sport to allow competition after injury; serious irreparable damage sometimes results. However, in most sports, their use is allowed by injection provided declaration of the use is made at the time of injection.

The control of doping in sport is based upon the unequivocal identification of the presence of a drug of one of the banned classes in a competitor but not the amount. The increasing sensitivity of tests presents a problem for medication by physicians using slowly eliminated drugs belonging to the banned classes, and it is advisable that such drugs should not be used within a week of competition.

On all of these above occasions, successful and unsuccessful challenges were based on the dissatisfaction of the athlete with the mechanism for testing positive for drug/dope substances. The battle between participants rightly and/or wrongly accused of taking banned substances and the international federations and domestic governing bodies for protecting the integrity of their particular athletic activities will no doubt continue. The emergence of new evidence concerning the apparent high level of state organized drug misuse among athletes in the former East Germany has already been noted. Prosecutions have followed. At the heart of the battles will be the observance of medical and para-medical practitioners of their ethical and legal responsibilities to their patients, *within the framework of the applicable sporting discipline.*

Every sporting discipline has its own criteria within the framework of the IOC guidelines.

It follows, almost without need for mention, that it is vitally important that every medical and paramedical practitioner should be aware of the regulatory requirements applicable to the appropriate sporting discipline within which their services are required when prescribing medicines.

Whenever possible, the medical and paramedical adviser should either attend or at a minimum be aware of the mechanism of drug testing procedures for his or her patient, and should be vigilant to observe that correct procedures are strictly observed. That said, the team doctor is unlikely personally to be able to check all stages of the storage transport of urine samples and transplant operations. The competence and integrity of governing bodies and laboratories is also paramount.

Finally, and importantly, consideration must be given to the little known reported US case of *Oksenholt v Lederle Laboratories* 656 Pacific Reporter 2d series 293 at 295–300 (1982). The Supreme Court of Oregen held that a physician, Erling Oksenholt, having prescribed a drug to a patient (not in a sporting context) who was subsequently blinded by the drug, was entitled to maintain an action for misrepresentation and negligence against the drug manufacturers. The grounds were that they had misrepresented or alternatively withheld information about the substance of the drug to the doctor: and certain foreseeable damages were recoverable as a result of that established misconduct (and if at the trial, the plaintiff's allegations of the defendant company's breach of duty and misrepresentation were established to have been made in deliberate disregard of the rights and welfare of others, they could also create a liability for punitive damages).

This is also a further dimension to the potential legal penalty area identified by Weiler and Roberts in their *Sports Law: Cases, Problems* cited in the Preface at pp. xxii–xxiii:

> Besides the team physician, an attractive third-party target for a tort suit by an injured player is the manufacturer of a product used in the game.

With the exploding growth of the international drug industry, this particular target area should not be ignored. Indeed, a further example comes from the valuable contribution of *Drug Distribution in the Training Room* in the *Clinics in Sports Medicine* series volume on *Sports Pharmacology* during July 1998, already cited at p. 40 (*supra*), on this occasion from Patsy Huff Pharm D, FASHP, at the University of North Carolina at Chapel Hill:

> Drug distribution is only one component of pharmaceutical care. The individual who provides pharmaceutical care assumes a degree of responsibility for the outcome of the patient. This liability was demonstrated in October, 1996, when a South Carolina court issued a judgment for more than $16 million against a pharmacy for negligence. The court found that the Plaintiff had incurred physical injuries, including brain damage, and suffered emotional trauma as a result of a dispensing error. The Plaintiffs also alleged that the employee failed to maintain proper policies and procedures for filling prescriptions. The individual providing pharmaceutical care for athletes needs to be knowledgeable in legal and regulatory issues related to medication distribution to reduce the risk of legal penalties, but more important, to reduce the risk of compromised care for athletes that might lead to averse patient outcomes: *Hundely-v-Rite Aid and Jones* (Court of Common Pleas, York County, South Carolina): 95-CB-46-405 and 406.

Chapter 6

# WMA Guideline 5

5   **The physician should inform the sportsman or athlete, those responsible for him, and other interested parties, of the consequences of the procedures he is opposing, guard against their use, enlist the support of other physicians and other organizations with the same aim, protect the sportsman or athlete against any pressures which might induce him to use these methods and help with supervision against these procedures.**

This particular guideline might have been formulated in more precise language. Its terminology suggests that a drafting lawyer was not involved in its creation or alternatively that it suffered in translation. Nevertheless it illustrates Sir Roger Bannister's earlier criteria cited in the Introduction: Why now – and how? (p. 15):

> Sports medicine encompasses cardiology, respiratory medicine, orthopaedic surgery, traumatology and many other specialities

and that the complexity of the subject, like sport itself, cannot be regarded in one dimension. Concurrently this emphasizes what is often overlooked or ignored by superficial commentators on the sporting legal scene, both within and without the legal profession. There is no jurisprudential subject of 'Sports law'. Comparable with sports medicine, it encompasses general legal principles applicable to sporting circumstances affecting different legal categories, from the conventional contract, crime and tort to patents, planning, tax and VAT as mere examples.

Whatever message can be spelt out from this Guideline, it can be seen at three different levels:

i    Basic recognized professional practice of informed consent;

ii   The recognized legal obligation to consult further;

iii  Avoidance of pressures which attempt to undermine authority of medical opinion as emphasized more specifically in Guideline 8 (see Chapter 8); and unaffected by third party interests.

For convenience of arrangement and simplicity, these three different levels can be dealt with most suitably in reverse order.

### iii  *Avoidance of pressures which attempt to undermine authority*

(a) This was illustrated vividly after the joint Football Association–Royal College of Surgeons (Edinburgh) joint Lilleshall Sports Medicine Conference on Sports Medicine and the Law was addressed by the writer. A doctor whose club the author had represented in relation to non-medical matters reversing an unjust Football League disciplinary decision enquired what he should do if ever his medical opinion were to be challenged by anyone, whether player, manager, coach or the Board of Directors. The answer that he should commit it to writing was endorsed by the FA chairman, and a former practising solicitor, Sir Bert Millichip, that it was 'the best advice you ever could give'.

At the time of writing on the 50th anniversary of the opening of the London Olympic Games on 29 July, 1948, no greater example exists beyond the unexplained substitution in the 1998 World Cup Football Final of the Brazilian Ronaldo after his initial exclusion from the team-sheet list because of an alleged injury, not yet identified officially. The true position has yet to emerge, administratively and clinically, if ever it will be told.

(b) In the American courts, the autonomy of medical care and opinion has been challenged in a comparable and similar context on a wider basis than in the UK. At present the US Supreme Court is reported to be asked to consider a pattern which has been unfolding since 1990; and clearly it is a developing scenario while athletes who are injured or risk prone because of an abnormality continue to claim a right to participate by reliance upon federal laws designed to protect the disabled.

(c) Two American statutes prohibit allegedly unjustified discrimination against people who have physical abnormalities or impairments. They do not render a physician liable for determining medical ineligibility, but they apply to virtually all professional teams and intercollegiate and interscholastic sports performances. (The Rehabilitations Act, 1973 and Americans with Disabilities Act, 1990.)

(d) In two US court decisions, the medical recommendations advising *against* participation in American football activities on evidence of high risk consequences did not violate the Rehabilitation Act (*Larkin v Archdiocese of Cincinnati*, No. C-1-90-619 (SD

OHIO, 31 August, 1990); *Pahulu v University of Kansas* 897 F Supp 1387 (D Kan 1995). In a third case, however, a federal court held that a university's exclusion of a player from its intercollegiate basketball programme, on the advice of the team's physician, breached the Rehabilitation Act; but a federal appeals court overruled the decision and decided that the team physicians do have the right in the patient's interest to bar athletes from competition for clear medical reasons. Nevertheless, the player's attorney has promised to appeal against the decision to the US Supreme Court *Knapp v Northwestern University*, No. 96-3450, US Ct of App 7th Cir, 22 November, 1996: See the *Physician and Sports Medicine*, October 1996, pp. 75–78; January 1997, pp. 19–20: an intention not reportedly altered at the time of writing in 1998; a disabled professional golfer invoked the ADA legislation to override playing restraints on his use of disability equipment for competition (*Martin v US PGA 1998*) Weiller Roberts, *Sports and the Law*, 2nd Edn, 1998, p. 876.

(e) On a wider medical basis than this sports related context, the UK courts have been invoked by doctors for authority to withdraw treatment, for example in circumstances of 'persistent vegetative state' (PVS) (see *Airedale NHS Trust v Bland* [1993] 1 All ER 821). In relation to a reverse situation, when medical authorities forced a Caesarian operation against a patient's will, the Court of Appeal granted leave to challenge the original decision later (see S's Application for judicial review, *Independent*, 10 July, 1997); and ultimately reported initially in the *British Medical Journal* for 16 May, 1998: p. 1480: Vol. 316 and later as *St George's Health NHS Trust v S* (1983) 3 WLR 936, the Court of Appeal (while laying down complex guidelines) re-affirmed the absolute right of a competent adult to refuse medical or surgical intervention, even if the result is certain death for herself or her foetus.

(f) Remaining with the UK sports scenario, legislation under the former Education Act 1944, s 76 (now s 9 of the Education Act 1996) has for over half a century been involved in attempts for children to be educated in accordance with the wishes of their parents, but hitherto in a non-sporting context beyond the scope of physical injuries which increase the risk to health of many sporting activities. The availability of this legislation in support of medical evidence, against the suitability of participation in potentially harmful sports activity, cannot be ignored or excluded, particularly in the light of the American and wider United Kingdom medicolegal recent court experiences.

*ii  Recognized legal obligation to consult further*

(a) *Wilson v Vancouver Hockey Club* (1983) 5 DLR (4th) 282 (BCSC) was another Vancouver hockey case where the defendant club was exonerated from liability because the doctor, although held to be negligent in his treatment, acted as an independent contractor and not as a servant of the club when he made the final decision as to what treatment an injured player should receive and whether he should play without advice from the club management. The doctor was in fact negligent because, although employed by the club to treat players for hockey injuries, he had failed to refer the plaintiff player for a biopsy on the player's arm to a specialist, even though he suspected the player to have a small skin cancer, which ultimately affected his playing career.

For a doctor acting as an independent contractor but skilfully in the interests of a player where *bona fide* medical opinion was challenged by the club, see *Keating v Tottenham Hotspur* (1997) *Times*, 17 July, 1997.

(b) Such liability is consistent with standard medical practice as summarized succinctly by Powers and Harris, 1900: 'Surgeons must be prepared to seek opinions on problems with which they deal only occasionally'.

In *Payne v St Helier Group Hospital Management Committee* [1952] CLYB 2442 the defendant casualty officer incorrectly diagnosed the abdominal injuries of a man who had been kicked by a horse. Donovan J held that the casualty officer was negligent in failing to have the man examined by a doctor of consultant rank.

In *R v Bateman* (1952) 94 lKB, Lord Hewart LCJ noted that 'it is no doubt, conceivable that a qualified man may be held liable for recklessly undertaking a case which he knew or ought to have known to be beyond his powers'. For a Canadian case in which a similar principle was applied see *Fraser v Vancouver General Hospital* [1951] 3 WWR (NS) 357 where a doctor was held to have been negligent in undertaking to interpret X-ray films, rather than referring them to an expert radiologist. Also from Canada, *MacDonald v York County Hospital* [1972] 28 DLR 521, cited at p. 40 in Chapter 1: Introduction for illustrating *res ipsa loquitor* affecting a foot amputation, was further negligent in failing to seek the advice or collaboration of a cardiovascular specialist. Furthermore, settlement was announced with an admission of liability that a former Olympic sprinter suffered severe brain damage following a road traffic accident because the initial diagnosis did not recognize initially the need for the subsequent specialist neurological services (*Cameron Sharp v North Cumbria Health Authority* (1997) *Daily Telegraph*, 18 February, *Guardian*, 20 February).

*i Basic recognized professional practice of informed consent*

This concept covers a wide area and is beyond sports medicine practice. To recall a controversial High Court verdict relating to neurological damage following a difficult aortography, *O'Malley-Williams v Board of Governors of the National Hospital for Nervous Diseases* (1975) cited in 1 BMJ 635 (see also Mason and McCall-Smith 4th edn p. 209) a plea of *res ipsa loquitur* was rejected on the grounds that the injury sustained was of a kind recognized as an inherent risk of the appropriate procedure. Nevertheless, Kennedy and Grubb in *Medical Law* (2nd edn, 1994) explained (p. 172) prior to a cascade of cases in the 1980s and 1990s which grappled with the problem generally:

> As the legal correspondent to the British Medical Journal commented, in discussing the *O'Malley-Williams* decision [(1975) 1 BMJ 635, 636]:
> [w]hether there is a positive duty on doctors to keep their patients informed of all aspects of their treatment, even when they pose no queries, is an issue of some importance to the [medical] profession and one that some day will have to be faced head-on.

As already cited in the Preface (p. xxv) from Kennedy and Grubb's later *Principles of Medical Law* (1998):

> The North American doctrine of 'informed consent' (always something of a misnomer) is not part of English law.

The USA scenario, however, is summarized conveniently by a contribution entitled *Legal Aspects of Sports Medicine* from Emidio Bianco and Elmer J. Walker (1994) in *Sports Medicine for the Primary Care Physician* (2nd edn, 1994) edited by Richard B. Birrer: CRC Press at p. 3:

1. Physician should explain nature of the procedure, treatment, or disease.
2. The patient should be informed about the expectations of the recommended treatment and the likelihood of success.
3. The patient should know what reasonable alternatives are available and what the probable outcome will be in the absence of any treatment.
4. The patient should be informed about the known inherent risks that are material to an informed decision about whether to accept or reject medical advice.

The converse of such consent which by medical standards can amount to fraudulent concealment is explained further there at p. 31 by Charles Krueger, a well-known defensive lineman with the

San Francisco Forty-Niners (49ers), who played college and professional football from 1955 until 1973 and had a history of multiple
left-knee injuries, which involved both ligaments and cartilage. He
received approximately 50 injections (Novocaine and cortisone) in
1964 and averaged 14 to 20 per year from 1964 until 1973.

At trial, Krueger charged the 49ers with fraudulent concealment
of medical information and alleged that he relied to his detriment
on the information that he received by continuing to play on a
severely damaged knee, that he would have retired rather than risk
progressive and permanent injury, and that the progressive and
permanent injuries to his left knee were the direct result of the team
physician's failure to fully disclose the nature of his injury and the
detrimental effects of continuing to play professional football. The
court observed that substantial evidence existed to show that the
team physician had failed to inform Krueger about the magnitude
of the risk he was taking by continuing to play professional football
on a damaged knee, and had failed to disclose the known adverse
affects of injecting corticosteroids into Krueger's left knee (234 Cal.
Rptr 579 (CA 1987)).

Finally, yet a further American source, *Law and the Team
Physician*: Elizabeth M Gallup (1955), claims in respect of the
earlier Vancouver hockey case (see also Ch 1 pp. 31–32 *supra*):

> Another case involving fraudulent concealment was the case of
> *Michael Robitaille v Vancouver Hockey Club*. In this case Robitaille,
> a hockey player, was hospitalized after suffering an injury to his
> shoulder and spinal cord. The team physicians concealed the true
> extent of his injuries, and the team later tried to trade him. The team
> to which he was traded discovered the extent of his injuries, and
> Robitaille subsequently sued with the damages award.

These issues add fuel to *British Medical Journal* commentary (see
p. 95 above) that there is an overriding issue beyond sports
medicine 'of some importance to the [medical] profession and one
that some day will have to be faced head-on'. If it has been faced
head-on beyond the realm of sports medicine, it clearly will require
head-on thinking when it exists in the context of a team unit and the
emergency illustrated by the Ronaldo selection or rejection as kick-
off time approached for the 1998 Football World Cup Final.

Chapter 7

# WMA Guidelines 6 and 7

**6**    **The sports physician has the duty to give his objective opinion on the sportsmen or athletes' fitness or unfitness clearly and precisely, leaving no doubt as to his conclusions.**

**7**    **In competitive sports or professional sports events, it is the physician's duty to decide whether the sportsman or athlete can remain on the field or return to the game. This decision cannot be delegated to other professionals or to other persons. In the physician's absence these individuals must adhere strictly to the instructions he has given them, priority always being given to the best interests of the sportsman's or athlete's health and safety, and not the outcome of the competition.**

These two Guidelines 6 and 7 supplement each other, with the medical practitioner entering centre stage

leaving no doubt as to his conclusions

(per Guideline 6) and

the best interests of the sportsman's health and safety, and not the outcome of the competition

(per Guideline 7).

The preamble to Guideline 7 also creates a two-dimensional level for:

1    The physician's direct decision.

2    The delegated responsibility to another for the physician in his or her absence.

The effect of either responsibility should be the same, whether direct or delegated, so far as it affects

the best interests of the sportsman's health and safety.

Nevertheless, the practical considerations involve the impact of any decision on:

1    Participants.

2   Organizations, including managers and coaches and sponsors.

3   Referees, umpires or other officiating sources.

4   The level of qualification of any delegated referral, e.g. at first-aid or physiotherapy level.

Each in turn can create an easily recognizable conflict with a medical opinion:

1   Participants may wish to continue or return to play against medical advice for preservation of a team selection or consideration for higher honours. (Frequently an unfit athlete rarely performs up to standard even for a limited period.)

2   Organizations or their personnel may wish to preserve a player's position for a comparable reason.

3   Referees or umpires or other officials may wish to preserve their authority without realizing that resisting medical advice could create a personal liability if a foreseeable injury occurs within the context of its particular sporting activity.

4   Delegated referrals with lesser experience and qualifications than physicians and surgeons, e.g. first-aiders and even sporting physiotherapists, and management and organizations MAY create tensions with more experienced and higher qualified practitioners.

These four practical criteria are illustrated by easily identified examples from the current international sporting scene, with its two-dimensional verbal and vision coverages at time of writing in 1998; and they must intensify and be repeated inevitably during and after publication of these pages.

1   Deal with participants and organizations which surfaced dramatically during the 1998 World Cup competition.

2   Referees' authority must always be linked to participatory safety, and

3   Delegated referrals and potential conflicts are likely to increase with the expansion of a universal *Sport for All Policy*.

Sample examples can be identified from the global scene generally, and USA and UK litigation court case precedents.

*1 Participatory wishes and medical advice*

During the 1998 World Cup Competition, under the headline 'England Playing Risky Game', Rob Hughes, the London *Times* Chief Sports Correspondent, alone apparently of his contemporaries identified under a subheading 'the danger that Michael Owen was left to endure'. It occurred during a goalkeeper collision in the preparatory fixture before competition began against Morocco. As Hughes wrote in depth for the issue of 29 May:

> Michael Owen's superb goal in Casablanca on Wednesday was undoubtedly the most valuable act of England's World Cup preparation. It emphasised what courage and desire, what pace and composure, he has. It will do the boy a power of good and his country needs that.
>
> However, that Owen was still on the field to score it was scary and irresponsible. Any parent of an 18-year-old, every neurologist who put his mind to what preceded it, would conclude that a player previously concussed should be removed from the danger of a second blow to the head.
>
> Owen, by his own admission, was knocked cold 25 minutes earlier when the knee of the Morocco goalkeeper, Driss Benzakri, caught his jaw. Dion Dublin took good care of his England colleague by turning him on his side and ensuring that the tongue had not been swallowed. Our players live and learn; Dublin has played for Manchester United where, in 1989, Bryan Robson swallowed his tongue.
>
> Owen quickly revived and appeared clear-eyed to the England doctor, John Crane. and two physiotherapists. "He didn't know what he was doing or what was happening," Glenn Hoddle, the coach, said. "But when he regained consciousness the first thing he did was plead not to be taken off, so we gave him another two minutes to recover his composure." Owen later admitted: "I might have told them I was OK, but I didn't feel OK."
>
> Whether two minutes, 25 minutes or 90 minutes, it constituted an unacceptable risk. Concussion is insidious. No one can look inside the skull and see brain damage, which is why boxers collapse in the night hours after being revived in the ring. Boxing, rugby and horse racing have long been unequivocal towards concussion: remove the participant and do not let him resume until expert opinion deems further repercussion to be unlikely.
>
> The last person to heed in the heat of the contest is a performer. Adrenalin overrules common sense. In Owen's eyes, the glory, and the chance to book his seat on the World Cup plane, was worth the risk. He was well aware that his goal makes him the youngest scorer in England team history – though one doubts he knows that Tommy Lawton, who set the previous record in 1938, ended his life after years of wretched migraines blamed on the knockouts that he took on active football service.
>
> We are, you see, a courageous nation. Bravery is perceived in the

image of Paul Ince in Rome last October, battling on, his head swathed in bandages. The blood seeping through was the red badge of courage, so terribly British. Curiously, Owen had his opportunity in Casablanca because Ian Wright, another forward whose swiftness is of prime importance, was withdrawn the instant he felt a hamstring pull. With injuries below the waist, England is stepping into line with sensible foreign precaution; above the neckline, we live dangerously in the past.

In 1974, FIFA, the world governing body, heeded the warnings and issued advice from its medical committee that even mildly concussed players should be substituted. The Football Association ignored the missive, paid only lip service to the offer of a leading London brain specialist, Andrew Lees, to investigate the hazards inherent in putting the head to the ball, the elbow or the boot. That specialist, and others, start from the opinion that it is beyond them to attempt to diagnose internal head damage in a few moments on a field surrounded by thousands of fans. "I might expect," one expert counselled, "to be sued if I gave the wrong advice and the player suffered."

With a career potentially as worthy as Michael Owen's, that knock-on risk is surely round the corner.

The position does not end there, however. A subsequent announcement explained, without a final conclusion, in more than one comment on the young player's insurable interest to at least his club, Liverpool, irrespective of his own personal interest, how:

> The cost of premiums to protect Michael Owen for £60 million could run into six figures, say The Association of British Insurers. Liverpool want to insure the 18-year-old for the huge sum, which is six times the cover they had for him last season.

Furthermore, a perceptive letter in the *Times* which endorsed Hughes' concern appeared a week later over the name and professional address of a practising solicitor with great medico-legal experience, Simon Eastwood, 35 Great Peter Street, Westminster, SW1 under the heading 'Safety Above All':

> Sir, Rob Hughes (May 29) was absolutely right to suggest that England had indeed played a risky game in allowing Michael Owen to stay on the field after suffering a bone-crunching collision with the Morocco goalkeeper in the recent international.
>
> All football supporters will understand the emotional drive that Hughes acknowledges in players at this level, and Owen's plea to stay on the field when questioned by the physiotherapist was completely predictable.
>
> The point is that the Football Association as the governing body responsible for the England team, has an overriding duty to ensure that proper procedures are in place to deal with these situations. The World Cup is, of course, the pinnacle for any footballer, but nothing can be more important than good health. The cost-benefit comparison

when we are looking at severe head injuries should overwhelmingly be resolved in favour of compulsory withdrawal from the field of play.

Hughes's observation about the lack of activity from the Football Association is accurate. The reference to concern by doctors in terms of giving the wrong advice is a problem leading increasingly to defensive medical strategies. These concerns emphasise the difficulty in focusing on crucial health issues even at the highest sporting level.

What is most important is to ensure systems are in place whereby participants in sporting activities, at whatever level, run the smallest possible risk of serious injury. All those involved in sport, and not just football, should learn the lesson from boxing, rugby and horse racing before it is too late.

The significance and value of this endorsement and Hughes' own perception cannot be emphasized too clearly. Earlier at the beginning of the year, 1998, a symposium was mounted by the Jockey Club in London, England, on the subject of concussion and head injuries in sport under the initiative of the well-known medical adviser, Dr Michael Turner. It had the advantage of expert specialist neurological opinions from as far afield as America (Robert Cantu), Australia (Paul McCrory) and London (Peter Hamlyn). They anticipated in clinical terms Hughes' analysis crystallized by Cantu and others as the *Second Impact Syndrome*. It was arguably identified in Hoddle's controversial book cited at the end of this chapter (p. 105). The problem is not new, but it is becoming identifiable with the initiative of the medical profession and commentators as enlightened as Rob Hughes. Not without significance, the fascinating and detailed informative *History of the Oxford University Association Football Club: 1872–1998* by one of its former captains, Colin Weir, and former schoolmaster at Lancing College and Sedburgh School, records how sixty years ago in the last season of 'Peace-time football before War came again', 1937–8:

> W.H. Pedley was expected to be centre-half, a good player very unlucky to miss his Blue when he was concussed just before the Varsity match, an injury which was believed later to have led to the brain tumour which killed him.

More recently this has echoes nearer our own time in the Oxford University rugby blue who died shortly after suffering a head injury during the course of play and resuming until collapsing, on the eve of that other Varsity match, at Twickenham, at the end of 1996.

## 2 Organizations' or personnel wishes to preserve a player's position

The Brazilian footballer Ronaldo's experience in the World Cup Final as interpreted by the London *Times* newspaper Dr Thomas Stuttaford, in the opening sentence of the Preface to these pages, can hardly be improved. It

> has excited as much comment as among sports enthusiasts

for both, the unanswered question at the time of writing is inevitably, what was the true reason behind the initial rejection from the team, and then the late selection?

The authentically recognized journal *Football Europe* summarized the issues in its 'World Cup Souvenir Special Edition' (August 1998):

> The first official team-sheet listed Edmundo in place of Ronaldo, who was said to be suffering from an ankle injury. Then, with barely 45 minutes to go before the first whistle, a second team-sheet was issued with Ronaldo re-instated. FIFA sources said the player had been given the all-clear to play by the hospital doctor. In reality Brazil coach Mario Zagallo had decided not to play Ronaldo, who had suffered nausea and headaches at the team hotel earlier in the day. Zagallo was over-ruled however, by Brazilian F.A. boss Ricardo Teixeira and by Ronaldo himself, who now insisted he was fit to play. ...
>
> As soon as play got under way, it was clear Ronaldo was not fit at all. At times he was struggling to walk, let alone run – though whether this was the result of physical injury or illness, or mental stress, we may never know.

A conclusion endorsed in the international journal *World Soccer*:

> We may never know the full story.

## 3 Referees' or umpires' authority conflicting with advice and forseeable injury

The traditional attitude of complete autonomy of playing officialdom which:

> disregards the best interests of the sportsmen's health and safety, and not the outcome of the competition

(per Guideline 7) can easily be identified as a classic example of Lord Acton' 5 well-worn concept:

> Power tends to corrupt, and absolute power corrupts absolutely.

The mythology and ill-informed beliefs among the unthinking sporting fraternities that the playing field or boxing ring are controlled exclusively by the referee or umpire unknown to the Rule of Law have long been dispelled by albeit grudging recognition that the law of the land does not stop at the touchline, boardroom or committee room. It also extends to health and safety, as the following sample cases demonstrate.

i   In the United Kingdom's landmark referee liability case of *Smoldon v Whitworth and Nolan* (1996) *Times*, 18 December (Ct App) arising from breach of the specific Laws of the Game to protect under-19 Colts players, a touch judge had alerted the referee specifically to a potential risk of injury, without any effective response, prior to the disastrous trauma suffered by the Plaintiff.

ii  Five years earlier on the occasion of the notorious self-inflicted injury by Paul Gascoigne when he tackled unlawfully a Nottingham Forest opponent in the 1991 FA Cup Final at Wembley Stadium, the distinguished orthopaedic surgeon John King, wrote to the *Times* (22 May) as Director of the Academic Department of Sports Medicine at the London Hospital Medical College:

> In certain contact sports such as rugby the referee has a duty to protect players from both others and themselves; a concussed player can be "sent off" by the referee and substituted.
> In the play on Saturday it is arguably clear that Mr Gascoigne was in a hyper-excited state as evidenced by his first tackle. Had the referee shown the yellow card it is most likely that the player would have modified his mood, especially given his world cup experience.
> This is not to say that the Hotspurs board should now sue the referee for their lost millions, but it is time to remind all arbitrators that they have a duty to protect players from damaging others and themselves.

iii From the USA with its differing and overlapping territorial jurisdictions the following are a specimen selection regularly cited in their transatlantic sources.

   (a) In *Mogabgab v Orleans Parish School Board* 239 So 2d 456 (La Ct App, 1970), an action was brought by parents for the wrongful death of their son, a high school football player who died as a result of heatstroke and exhaustion following a practice. The plaintiff sued the coach, the school principal, and the school district for the allegation that the school was negligent in not making sure the coach was properly trained.

They argued that the school was negligent in making arrangements for the proper care of sick and injured players. The court held that the coach, who actively denied student access to medical treatment for two hours after symptoms of heatstroke and shock appeared, was guilty of negligence. It did not find negligence attributable to the principal, school district, physical education supervisor, or school superintendent, however, because they were either unaware of the events or on vacation.

(b) In *Stineman v Fontbonne College* 664 F 2d 1082 (8th Cir, 1981), an action was brought by Patricia Stineman, a deaf student who had played on the Fontbonne College softball team. Her softball coaches were aware of her deafness. Stineman had also signed an authorization for emergency medical treatment in the event of an injury. During the course of practice, plaintiff was struck in the eye with a ball. Although she was in great pain, a coach merely applied ice and advised Stineman to go to her room and rest. Neither of the coaches who were present suggested that she seek medical attention. No immediate professional medical attention was given, even though the school infirmary was across the street. Permanent eye damage resulted from the injury. The trial court awarded Stineman $800 000 in damages for the negligence of the defendant in failing to provide medical assistance. The Court of Appeals affirmed the decision, finding the college vicariously liable; however, the court reduced the award to $600 000.

N.B. This also can be cited as a further illustration of Chapter 6: WMA Guideline 5, and its requirement to consult further (p. 91 *supra*).

(c) In *Benitez v New York City Board of Education* 541 NE 2d (NY Ct App, 1989) a high school football player sued the local board of education and city public school athletic league, alleging negligence against the coach and principal for permitting his participation in a mismatched game whilst in a fatigued condition. An appellate court exonerated the Defendants on the basis that the Plaintiff assumed the risks of injury and was not under inherent compulsion to play. Fatigue, concussion, diabetes, dehydration and cold are all factors here.

(d) Marc Buoniconti was the linebacker for a college football team. He suffered a series of neck injuries in consecutive games and was allowed to participate in contact games drills during the week prior to a game in which he suffered a paralysing injury. A jury acquitted the doctor from a negligence claim on the basis of full assumption of risk by the player, although an issue relating to fitness of product liability concerning a face mask strap was also raised, with an ultimate out-of-court settlement (Berry and Wong (1993), p. 511).

## 4 Delegate referrals

An example of the tensions which can lie concealed beneath the surface emerged during a high profile, interesting but inconclusive dispute between the Tottenham Hotspur Football Company Club and one of its medical advisers, Dr Patrick Keating. An industrial tribunal claim for unfair dismissal was rejected, as reported in the *Times*, the *London Evening Standard* and the *British Medical Journal* on the basis of no contract of employment. The doctor was found to have been engaged as an independent contractor who had been paid fees rather than a salary. The allegation of non-referral of a star player to specialist services was rejected by the club (see *British Medical Journal* Vol. 315: 903, 11 October, 1997). What does not appear from any of these four reported citations is whether or not the Canadian case of *Robitaille v Vancouver Ice Hockey Club* (*supra*) was referred to. Certainly it is not cited in any of the traditional medical legal negligence United Kingdom authorities apart from a negative reference in Kennedy and Grubb in *Medical Law* (1994) on the issue of contributory negligence.

Assessment by the English courts must be awaited, bearing in mind that Ontario courts relied on the British precedent and the element of control in *Morren v Swinton and Pendelbury Borough Council* [1965] 2 AER 349 at 351 (see Chapter 1: *Sport and the law in the world of medicine* at p. 21 *supra*).

## CONCLUSION

It is worth recording that the categories of potential negligence and liability are never closed. The issues inherent in the factual content of this chapter are too serious to be ignored by all concerned at every level of sport and exercise medicine. The facts contained in the graphic photograph and caption between pages 128 and 129 of *My 1998 World Cup Story*, by Glenn Hoddle and David Davies, provide a textbook example to debate them. Michael Owen 'was out cold for a few seconds and his first words as he came round were "I don't want to come off"'. He went on to score the winner'.

Chapter 8

# WMA Guidelines 8, 9 and 10

**8   To enable him to carry out his ethical obligations the sports physician must see his authority fully recognized and upheld, particularly wherever it concerns the health, safety and legitimate interests of the sportsman or athlete, none of which can be prejudiced to favour the interests of any third party whatsoever.**

**9   The sports physician should endeavour to keep the patient's personal physician fully informed of facts relevant to his treatment. If necessary he should collaborate with him to ensure that the sportsman or athlete does not exert himself in ways detrimental to his health and does not use potentially harmful techniques to improve his performance.**

**10  In sports medicine, as in all other branches of medicine, professional confidentiality must be observed. The right of privacy over medical attention the sportsman or athlete has received must be protected, especially in the case of professional sportsmen or athletes.**

These criteria highlight the potential minefield in which a sports practitioner can be trapped. They apply equally to amateur as well as to professional participants.

Furthermore, they can create a potential conflict of medical responsibility if the sportsperson's or athlete's medical condition discloses a condition which the patient may not wish to be disclosed to his 'personal physician', particularly if that would affect the sportsperson's employer–employee relationship extraneous to sporting activity (for example, a concussed lorry driver, injured during a sporting fixture). The dilemma posed by this conflict can arise between a doctor's confidentiality duty to the patient and a contractual employment, or even a governmental imposed statutory commitment within an overriding positive duty framework.

The conflict and dilemma within a sporting context has been illustrated in a recent citation involving law and employment.

In *Baker v Kaye* (1996) *Times*, 13 December [1997] IRLR 214 a potential employee failed to establish negligence against a company doctor who had examined the candidate and did not recommend employment. Subsequently, in *Kapfunde v Abbey National and Anor* (1988) CAT 98-0495, the Court of Appeal rejected any duty found in *Baker v Kaye* by an employer or insurer commissioned doctor to a potential employee, and also queried, in such circumstances, the existence of a doctor–patient relationship.

Athletes will not seek help or advice from a team physician whom they cannot trust to keep their confidence – regardless of whether they want advice about performance-enhancing drugs or other, no less sensitive matters. One area, however, in which this has yet to be resolved will emerge when a competitor-patient discloses a transmissible infectious condition, and particularly that of HIV and/or HBV (hepatitis B virus). In the British Medical Association *ABC of Sports Medicine* (1995), the contribution on '*Infections*' by J. C. M. Sharp, one of the honorary medical advisers to the Scottish Rugby Union, explains that at that time [p. 32]:

> With one apparent exception [an Italian soccer player: documented in the UK *Lancet*, 1990: Vol. 1: 1105], there remains to date no evidence worldwide of the transmission of either HIV or HBV infection while participating in sport. Cuts or abrasions during sporting activity clearly require attention and bleeding to be controlled before players return to the field of play. ... More recently the International Rugby Football Board has prepared guidelines specific to bloodborne infections and contact sports.

A year prior to that disclosure, a joint medico-legal contribution from Australia in the *Monash University Law Review* (1994, Vol. 20, p. 214) from Roger S. Magnusson and Hayden Opie identified high-profile international sports participators who had admitted their personal contamination, and explained:

> Many sports have been stimulated to develop and implement infectious diseases policies. This has led to questions of a legal nature being raised about these policies. Many of the legal issues raised are entirely novel, and until the courts and Parliaments deal with them specifically, it will be a case of taking general principles and the experiences gained in other contexts and adapting them to the circumstances of sport.

Five sample experiences in the courts and in line with the issues raised in *Baker v Kay*, but with differing results, can be seen from two American sports-related decisions, and one or more general principles consistent with them, from the United Kingdom.

In *Chuy v Philadelphia Eagles Football Club* 431 F Supp 254 (ED Pa 1977); *affd* 595 F 2d 1265 (3rd Cir, 1979), the plaintiff, a former professional football player, sought damages from his club for 'intentional infliction of emotional distress'. The court held that there was sufficient evidence to support the jury's determination that the team physician had intentionally or recklessly inflicted mental distress on the plaintiff. The physician had made a false statement to the press about a supposedly fatal disease from which the plaintiff was suffering. The club was held vicariously liable for the physician's breach of confidentiality. Nevertheless, the court held that the Eagles football club had the right to control and did control the substance of the team's statements to the press concerning physical conditions of its athletes.

Physicians, however, may have a duty to warn third parties of impending harm related to an athlete's drug use, and a team physician's public duty to warn may override the private duty of confidentiality. Anabolic steroids are known to cause personality changes and heighten aggressiveness and may cause law-abiding and psychiatrically asymptomatic individuals to develop manic and psychotic symptoms – culminating occasionally in criminality. Physicians must properly consider reporting patients who develop such tendencies.

This duty was illustrated in 1990 after a physician had prescribed steroids to a police officer attempting to get into shape for the police Olympics. The officer developed a steroid-induced psychosis, became violent, and shot three individuals. Within a complex procedural framework the Indiana Court of Appeals heard that the appellant physician had overmedicated the patient with anabolic steroids and testosterone to the point that he became a toxic psychotic and thereby imminently dangerous to third persons. On a further appeal, the Supreme Court of Indiana held it was *not* possible to foresee (within a negligent context) when the officer was likely to attack the victim and thus the doctor had no duty to warn the victim that she was in danger of physical harm (*Webb v Jarvis* 575, NE 2nd 992 Ind. 1991). A few months earlier, on this side of the Atlantic, an English Court of Appeal upheld disclosure of an independent psychiatrist report to a hospital where a plaintiff was detained, urging the hospital to forward a copy to the Home Secretary, on the basis that public interest in disclosure outweighed the patient's private interest (*W v Edgell* [1990] Ch 359).

Finally, in the television media-dominated global village in which all alleged public entertainment sport exists today, the risk of breach of confidence can be substantial and the consequences formidable. Thus, in mid-1997, a sequence of press reports from hospital sources about an alleged drug overdose by a well-known fashion model were refuted by her legal advisers in circumstances which subsided as rapidly as they had surfaced. In the present commercial climate of sponsored athletes doubling as fashion models and at times today claiming the need for counselling, this particular ethical territory will require careful monitoring by all associated with public prudence in the health and sickness of *public performers* on every stage, as distinct from the more robust participators at the grass roots levels of healthy education-recreational fun and joy and pleasure.

Further, this catchment area of liability is not confined exclusively to the medical profession. A little known decision of the USA District Court of Ohio in *Hammonds v Aetna Casualty and Surety Co.* 243 F.Supp 793 (N.D. Ohio 1965) affirmed procedurally a patient's right to sue the doctor's insurer for allegedly inducing the doctor to divulge confidential information given through the false pretext that the plaintiff was contemplating a malpractice suit. A decade later in the USA, the better known citation of *Tarasoff v Regents of California* (1976) 551 P2d 334 established liability by a student medical centre for failing to warn a young woman of the risk posed to her by one of their patients who, ultimately, murdered the girl. It had failed to breach their patient's confidence and warn the girl of the threat to her life, which had been confessed to a therapist at the centre, who had even warned the police.

Finally, in the United Kingdom at least, separate from whatever may exist elsewhere, Parliament has imposed mandatory statutory compulsion for disclosure of what ordinarily would be confidential information and material. This includes reporting of infectious diseases, industrial injuries and diseases and registration of drug addicts.

Significantly, in the context of Guideline 9 and the global interest in the Ronaldo-Brazil-World Cup mystery, the ever-informative BBC World Service Sports programme broadcasting to the world at 03.15 hours Greenwich Mean Time reported on Wednesday 15 July after the competition had ended that Ronaldo's Italian club, Inter Milan, had said it was not worried by accounts that the 21-year-old Brazilian may have been too stressed to play in the final round of the competition won by France. An Inter spokeswoman, Susannah Wermelinger, explained 'he is a well-balanced individual' and also that the club had been in close contact with him during the World Cup. His subsequent return to form and fitness by the end of 1998 confirmed that mature assessment.

Chapter 9

# WMA Guidelines 11 and 12

**11  The sports doctor must not be party to any contract which obliges him to reserve particular forms of therapy solely and exclusively for any one sportsman or athlete or group of sportsmen or athletes.**

**12  It is desirable that sports physicians from foreign countries, when accompanying a team in another country, should enjoy the right to carry out their specific functions.**

These two guidelines may not appear to have an immediate direct connection. Nevertheless, a moment's reflection can indicate how a team group or tour, whether at home or overseas, can lend itself to priority demands for urgent treatment of whatever medical kind.

Within that framework it is hoped that it would be inconceivable that any responsible medical or paramedical practitioner would give, under contract, preferential treatment for any particular patient, whatever may be the temptation because of personal or professional associations. If the Munich disaster were sadly to be repeated today, any contractual prohibition upon a German club doctor creating a local exclusivity to prevent his assisting the English team would be a breach of Guideline 11. At the time of writing there were no known cases of such an accusation against a doctor. Very few of the many books dealing with sports injuries and/or medicine generally deal with the team doctor and paramedical associates, whether nationally or internationally.

Three sources to be cited hereafter which are United Kingdom based, are nevertheless applicable internationally; underlying every circumstance for 'accompanying a team in another country', on the international sports circuit is the desirability (and indeed necessity) for obtaining legal advice, and the opportunity to apply for medico-legal indemnity insurance against professional negligence in any part of the world through the appropriate protection societies or defence unions. However, the perceived wisdom is that this is unlikely to be obtainable if at all, unless at prohibitive expense, for the US and Canada, from where so many of the legal precedents within this text have emerged.

The most comprehensive summary generally for the role of sports physicians 'when accompanying a team in another country' is that provided by Donald Macleod, the Honorary Medical Adviser to the Scottish Rugby Unions, President of the BASM. It appears in the BMA *ABC of Sports Medicine* (1995) pp. 57–58 where he explains that:

> A doctor and chartered physiotherapist usually make up the staff involved in the medical care of a team but this can vary between sports and many include a masseur or sports scientist. The essential difference between team medical care and colleagues providing services at an event or to a governing body in sports is the very special, professional but highly committed and enduring relationship that arises as the result of being part of the inner circle of players, coaches, selectors, and the team manager.

| Sports medicine supports sport |
|---|

| Player<br>Coach     Officials<br>Medical team |
|---|

| Medical | | Scientific |
|---|---|---|
| Diagnostic<br>Therapeutic<br>Rehabilitation | | Nutrition<br>Physiology<br>Psychology |

The medical team aims to underpin the playing team and must therefore be an integral part of the inner circle if they hope to provide the highest standards of occupational health.

The medical team cannot expect to be omnicompetent in the increasingly sophisticated world of sports medicine and sports science. The team will require appropriate facilities as well as a network of specialist advisers.

The medical team shares the highs and lows of their teams successes and failures as well as working with individuals to help them to achieve their peak performance. To this end, the medical team should set realistic objectives.

In most sport the medical team may well be giving their professional advice on a voluntary basis but this does not allow for any lowering of professional standards of practice – players are not experimental preparations or second class citizens.

The performing life of an athlete may be very short and the pressures to compete are intense but the medical team must be objective about the individual player/patient while remaining enthusiastically committed to the players and their realistic goals.

The medical team must demonstrate many personal and professional skills if they are to win a respected position in the inner circle. Members of the medical team must work together to fulfil their respective roles, clarifying lines of communication. There is no place for prima donnas in the medical team. Mutual respect and support are essential.

If it is to fulfil its role in the inner circle, the medical team must work with a wide range of officials. These include coaches, selectors, and managers, referees, and administrators. They should also clarify the exact professional relationship between the players, their general practitioners, and officials. In contacts with the media and the public the medical team should maintain clinical confidentiality and ethical standards, with no discussion of patient details without permission.

Donald Macleod's counterpart from the Scottish Football Association, W. Stewart Hillis, Professor of Cardiovascular and Exercise Medicine, developed this more recently in the *British Journal of Medicine* under the heading of 'Preparations for the World Cup', 1988, 32:55:

Every four years a great challenge occurs for medical officers to national football associations.

Preparation for this [1998] competition has required the interaction of administrators, coaches, and the medical support team. Organisational requirements comprise the standard tasks of choice of hotel and additional facilities, acclimatisation for climatic conditions, the individual preparation of players, and provision of first aid treatment and further medical facilities when required in the case of injury or illness.

A Scottish medical staff comprising two doctors, three physiotherapists, and one masseur will prepare the 22 players. If deemed necessary, separate nutritional and psychological advice will be provided. Each backroom staff member has a special role, but the medical group meet daily each morning to discuss all problems so that the whole group is aware of any problems raised to one of their members. Although managing elite footballers who make up the international squad will be personal, it obviously requires both individual and group support. Our approach is complementary to their standard preparation and additional to their personal requirements. Standard times for examination and treatment are arranged and appointments made for massage. Each player has had standard haematological and biochemical screening and standard cardiological and respiratory assessments. They have been given advice about doping in sport, and general lectures on the treatment and avoidance of injury and infection control and management. A detailed proforma of their nutritional preparation, standard form of fluid intake, and prophylactic treatment, such as strappings, has been obtained by questionnaire.

Contact has been made with the local organising committee at each venue, particularly the medical coordinating office and the local liaison doctor. A submission has been made to allow our two doctors to practise medicine in France, and detailed customs declarations have been submitted to allow for the free entry of our medical drugs and equipment. Details of the basic first aid provision at each match venue have been reviewed and the appropriate medical support contacted for both training and match venues. Local contact has been made with hospitals and other support services in each locality.

Consistent with these Scottish experiences, the England Football Association and Arsenal team doctor, John Crane MB ChB, wrote under the heading of 'Association football: the team doctor' in *Medicine, Sport and the Law* (Blackwell: 1990, p. 337):

When the national side travels abroad it is usual to make arrangements for a local orthopaedic surgeon to be available at the game, to help with the acute management of any severe injury during play. I usually contact the British Orthopaedic Association before leaving the UK to find an orthopaedic surgeon from the country to be visited. Immunisations to cover foreign travel is the responsibility of the team doctor. He must also attain up-to-date knowledge of the conditions of the environment which the team might have to encounter. Altitude, high temperatures and humidity are such conditions. Acclimatisation is important.

This general practitioners' experience was also emphasized by Malcolm Bottomley, the medical officer to the British athletes team in an accompanying chapter 'Athletes at an overseas venue: the role of the team doctor' from the same source at p. 163:

The professional relationship that exists between the team doctor and the athletes is akin to that of a factory medical officer and its employees, although, when abroad, the function is extended since the doctor also has to act as the 'GP'.

Finally, in a valuable comprehensive publication under the title of *The Team Physician's Handbook* from the other side of the Atlantic, under the following legal and medico-legal summarized caption headings, Morris B. Mellion and Michael Walsh (1990) explained at pages 5 and 6, but without any further textual expansion relating to medico-legal issues throughout the book:

*Legal and medico-legal*
1. Contract with school, league, or team.
2. Permission to treat minors.
3. Liability (a) institutional liability (b) professional liability.
4. Athlete's right to participate.
5. Treatment of athletes on out-of-state trips.

(a) Legality.
(i) For major athletic events the host state or country generally passes legislation granting visiting team physicians temporary licenses.
(ii) For routine competitions and tournaments it is recommended that the travelling team physician work through the host team or tournament physician or local physician in the host town.
(b) 'Good Samaritan' laws.
(i) No suit has yet been brought against a team player travelling with a team to another state over the issue of practising without a license.
(c) Professional liability insurance coverage.

This last requirement of insurance coverage is applicably equally for recreational players of all ages and in all circumstances. In the United Kingdom a developing awareness among regional as well as national governing bodies of their responsibility to alert their members to this is unfolding, and the Middlesex and Sussex County Football Associations are in the vanguard of this area. Because so many sports administrators and organizations worldwide function on an amateur and voluntary basis, the general absence of any coherent or structured guidance in this crucial health and injury protection circumstance is hardly surprising.

Furthermore, the criteria for insurance cover in relation to sports medical practitioners at all levels in the growing climate of American-induced litigation can also require special provisions such as evidence of capacity and qualifications and even access to the necessary equipment and back-up facilities.

Additionally, from the other side of the Atlantic during the final stages of proof correction yet a further contribution from the USA entitled *Team Physician or Athlete's Doctor?* from Dr Aaron Rubin, Director of the Kaiser Permanent Sports Medicine Fellowship in Fontana, California, and a member of the editorial board of *The Physician and Sports Medicine*, crystallized the tensions which have yet to be faced by not only the medical world generally, but also the whole ethos of sport at every level. Writing as a High School doctor he explained (July 1998: Vol. 26, No. 7):

> If a team is defined as any group organized to work together, then there's no doubt the team physician is on the team. We're part of the group, working towards a mutual goal. But what is that goal? Most of the time it seems the uppermost thing in the minds of the players and coaches is winning, and that's understandable. But team physicians can't afford to buy the idea that winning is "the only thing". If we do, we are putting winning ahead of the athletes' health. We need to remember that team sports are also about having fun, learning teamwork, and building fitness.

He also raised an issue which is almost inevitable with the emergence of the high profile within the current sporting social milieu by explaining further at page 28:

> Given the nature of a team physician's responsibilities, it concerns me that some physicians are now willing to "buy" positions with professional teams in order to boost their own reputation. I foresee a day when similar activity could take place with college teams and at other levels.
>
> Those few I know who are involved in this are excellent physicians and, as far as I know, give very good care, but it concerns me that the blurry line between team physician and athlete's protector becomes more distinct as the business of sports medicine becomes the driving force. Will physicians motivated by increased visibility really put the athletes' best interests first? We in sports medicine must determine ethical standards for this and other situations before others legislate the standards.

Dr Rubin wrote without any apparent awareness of the WMA Guidelines. Adherence to them throughout the world will avoid the need for any such legislation.

Chapter 10

# WMA Guideline 13

**13 The participation of a sports physician is desirable when sports regulations are being drawn up.**

The source of inspiration for such medical practitioner-led regulations will frequently be a combination of circumstances identifying a gap to be filled, and the initiative will often come from sports medical sources, who alert administrators to existing or anticipated dangers with the aim of preventiing injury.

In the UK, such circumstances surfaced during a power boating fatality when a hydroplane collided with a gas ferry jetty at Bristol docks, in 1986. A Royal Yachting Association (RYA) board of inquiry included the RYA honorary medical officer and recommended removal of the jetty and other safety actions, which actions were affirmed by the avoidance of similar consequences a year later on the occasion of a similar accident.

During the 1992 World Cup cricket competition the English cricket authorities were criticized for allowing the players to tour without a full-time medical practitioner. The medical adviser to the Essex County Cricket Club, Dr Tom Crisp, Mr John King, FRCS the director of the Department of Sports Medicine at the London Hospital Medical College, Tom McNab, a leading athletic ICS coach, and John Brewer, the head of the Human Performance Centre at the FA's Sports Medicine Institute at Lilleshall, were unanimous in their condemnation of absence of such services, notwithstanding the presence of an experienced physiotherapist (*The Times*, 21 March, 1992). In due course this gap was filled, with medical as well as physiotherapist services accompanying English cricket touring teams today; and thereby in a position to identify for the game's administrators such breaches of the Laws of the Game likely to endanger health and risk injury in the spirit contemplated by this Guideline 13.

Indeed, in following the *Smoldon* rugby referee negligence judgments (Curtis J and Court of Appeal: see p. 22 *supra*) the various cricket authorities concerned with regulating the Laws of the Game, the MCC, who possess their copyright, the National Cricket

Association (NCA), the Test and County Cricket Board and the Association of Cricket Umpires and Scorers, collectively sought legal advice for tightening up umpires responsibilities for observing applications of the laws of the game in relation to safety precautions to poor light; generally poor conditions; fast, short pitched bowling; and fast, high, full pitched bowling. The ultimate sanction of any changes in cricket's laws devolved upon the International Cricket Council (ICC) as well as requiring ratification by the MCC. Such public announcements which have accompanied the proposals did not include citations from medical or paramedical sources: but the focus on the changes for safety of players inferentially incorporates the consequences of the *Smoldon* judgment in its wider implications to risk management sport officials generally.

Rugby Union football in particular has been influenced responsibly by its medical advisers. The celebrated judgment in the schoolboy's unsuccessful claim for alleged negligent coaching and non-insurance, in *Van Oppen v Bedford School Trustees* (see p. 72, *supra*) resulted from a Medical Officers of Schools Association (MOSA) report in 1979 which recommended compulsory insurance for all rugby playing schools.

As a result of the conference of rugby union doctors, which did not include an International Rugby Football Board (IRFB) representative, in the context of increased competition from an admittedly physical game, a ten-point list of recommendations was formulated for the IRFB, as at 1991. In the intervening seven years they have all been implemented:

Recommendations of the Bermuda Conference

1 Referees, coaches and teachers and other non-playing designates to have certified training in first aid, including cardiopulmonary resuscitation (CPR) and the recognition of concussion.

2 That referees should be compelled to ensure that the current laws are adhered to by players at all levels of the game and most especially at the highest level and where players' safety is at risk.

3 Conference has verified the high incidence of injuries to the tackler and ball carrier, and these include the high incidence of brain and neck injuries. The safe and correct technique in tackling and failing by coaches and teachers must be re-emphasized.

4 Rugby injury surveys to be standardized as a matter of urgency according to a common protocol and nomenclature under the International Rugby Board (IRB).

5 *IRB Resolution 5.7* which states that a player who has suffered definite concussion 'should not participate' in any match or training for a period of at least 3 weeks from the time of the injury, and then only subject to being cleared by a proper neurological examination. The 'should not participate' to be reworded to '*must* not participate'.

6 Conference has identified the high incidence of injuries due to foul play and emphasized the responsibility and civil and criminal legal liability of rugby authorities. Foul play *must* be severely punished and the frequent offender must not be selected.

7 Civil liability incurred by doctors providing their professional services in the management of rugby injuries was identified by the Conference as a significant risk to practitioners, especially where services are provided in, or around a match situation: playing, training or touring. Ethical dilemmas within the doctor–patient relationship arising from the possibility of an ambiguous allegiance between the doctor, his patient and the club, were also considered. The IRB is called upon to clarify (and regularize) the relationship between the team and its medical attendant and to make adequate provision for professional indemnity arrangements where necessary.

8 The IRB *forthwith* should develop, agree and advertise to all members and associate member unions, rules including penalties and sanctions relating to the use and abuse of drugs and prohibitive substances. Conference recommended that the IOC guide-lines be adhered to.

9 Conference confirmed the potential risk of the transferral of hepatitis B virus and HIV. Players must not be allowed to compete with open bleeding wounds which cannot effectively be covered by an impermeable dressing.

*Note.* Contagious lesions such as scrumpox are included in this recommendation.

10 Conference identified the risk of febrile illness specifically affecting the cardiovascular system. Players who are ill or febrile *must not* be allowed to compete.

In 1991 Professor Michael Garraway, Donald Macleod, and Dr J. C. M. Sharpe published 'Rugby injuries devised for case registers' in the *BMJ* and four years later in the *Lancet*, vol 345:1485 (10th June) under the title of 'Epidemiology for rugby football injuries', Professor Michael Garraway and Donald Macleod (the latter in his capacity of honorary physician of the Scottish Rugby Union) (Garraway and MacLeod, 1995) expressed their purpose to report 'the frequency, nature of circumstances and outcome of rugby injuries in a prospective cohort consisting of virtually all players registered with senior clubs in the South of Scotland District of the Scottish Rugby Union'.

The report produced an encouraging response in the comment and correspondence pages of the *Lancet* at that time. Its work is still in progress and demonstrates the demand and need for the role of medicine in all sport to create a factual foundation towards the presentation and rehabilitation of victims in injury in sport.

More recently an end-of-year survey during Christmas 1997 from the distinguished and experienced *Times* rugby correspondent,

Gerald Davies, commented adversely on the insidious infiltration of the permission in rugby union football:

> ... to wear shoulder pads. It is but a short step to allow harder and tougher material of the kind American footballers wear. When one wonders, will helmets arrive on the scene?
>   What motivates the changes? Is it truly for the protection of the players or is it the case that, by agreeing such protection, the rugby union authorities can allow their game to become more powerful and more confrontational?

A response from Donald Macleod with the authority and experience from his position as Honorary Medical Adviser to the Scottish Rugby Union and President of BASM appeared a week later to endorse Davies' apprehensions and explain that protective padding was to be discussed at the IRFB's Medical Advisory Committee; and at the time when these pages go to press this crucial development for players' safety and avoidance of injury is still under review.

In a different dimension, a valuable insight illustrative of this regulatory guidance appeared in the London *Evening Standard* at the time of the 1997 All England Lawn Tennis and Croquet Club's Wimbledon Championship under the pen of Rhys Williams (June 27) subtitled 'On the million dollar girls and the tightrope they walk on the demanding tennis circuit'. Dealing with the relatively tender age of the media-targeted starlets, and the burn-out syndrome (see p. 62, *supra*) Rhys Williams explained how, partly at the instigation of Pam Shriver, then President:

> The WTA convened a commission to study the rules, comprising seven medical and sports science professionals. They solicited oral and written testimonies from players, former players, parents, coaches, agents, sponsors to get some picture of the pressures on tour and decide how best to equip young players to deal with them. 'The number one stress was the media', says Kathleen Stroia, a commissioner and director of sport science and medicine for the WTA. 'What that means is questions like "how do I best handle a Press conference" and "what happens if there's a negative article?"' Other common pressures, Stroia says, included pushy or demanding parents and loneliness. Capriati, Jaeger, who now runs a cancer foundation, and Gabriela Sabatini all contributed. "Their comment and feedback have been enormously valuable" says Stroia. The upshot was that in 1995, the age eligibility rules, which had allowed 14 year olds to play on an unrestricted basis were amended. A 14 year old may now play only five professional events a year, a 15 year old up to nine. At 16, it rises to 14 and increases to 18 at the age of 17. Unrestricted play now begins at 18. Critics of the new rules say that sane, responsible, talented young players are having to pay for the waywardness of

others. That the WTA has framed absurdly constricting regulations to assuage its guilt over the apparent failure to act earlier. Stroia says that the rules have just been implemented and are up for discussion. But she also makes the point that while some young players are not happy, they will thank the WTA when they are still playing and earning in 10 years time.

Certainly, the WTA has acted within the spirit, as well as the letter, of this WMA guideline.

Every sporting governing body with a risk element contained within it should be aware of the need to provide its own medical resources for the purpose expressed by this guideline. The high-risk activities from the worlds of horse and motor racing, boxing and rugby union football, whose ongoing medical services are perpetually in action, demonstrate its purpose. If it might have been thought to be superfluous, the examples provided here suggest that it is not. Indeed, while these pages were in preparation, a classic instruction emerged of how the concern for safety extends beyond a particular sport and its governing body. Notwithstanding the scrupulously careful safety criteria imposed by Fédération Internationale du Sport Automobile (FISA), under its English barrister president Max Mosley, the death of Ayrton Senna inspired criminal proceedings which eventually were resolved in the Italian courts. The Italian Olympic National Committee, with the patronage of the European Olympic Committees, mounted a Congress entitled 'Guilty of Wanting to Win: Penal Liability in Sports Activity'. The initiative expressly intended to 'clarify which are the liabilities connected with the organization of events for risky sports, as there are no uniform regulations in that field in the various countries.

The UK's delegate, Sir Maurice Drake, who had been the trial judge in the landmark case of *Elliott v Saunders and Liverpool Football Club*, a civil trial for changes, arising from serious ligament injuries, explained the UK differences between civil and criminal criteria for proof of guilt to wants victory, and other delegates displayed comparable enlightened explanations for the mechanisms of how the law operates to protect and prevent victims from sporting malpractices. Nevertheless, the world of medicine is in the front line for tending to the wounded from playing violence and always in the battles to want victory, and in the light of the belated recognition by the FA in August 1997 because of its concern regarding the growing list of casualties, it set up the medical research which will contact the physiotherapy departments of all Premier and Football League Clubs (*Daily Telegraph*, 4 August, 1997). It is worth recalling the pioneering analytical assessments of

Dr John Silver at Britain's National Spinal Injuries Centre at Stoke Mandeville in Buckinghamshire, J. P. R. Williams, John Davies (now Professor) and Terry Gibson (respectively in South Wales and Guy's Hospital, London) of the consequences, in rugby, of collapsing scrums and deliberate violent foul play (Williams and McKibbin; Davies and Gibson, 1978).

Chapter 11

# Guidelines – Summary

Looking back at the WMA's guidelines, what emerges from the earlier analysis by Donald Macleod in *The Doctor's Contribution Towards Safety in Sport* is their incompleteness in one respect. They have been overtaken by the culture gap between the professional entertainment world of sport and its existence for health and education, within or without competition. He has explained in *Medicine, Sport and the Law* (Blackwell, 1990) how doctors involved in sport have an ethical and legal duty to provide competent professional services and to ensure that they practise to a high standard with appropriate facilities – for example, National Health Service standards and facilities and he claims:

> The doctor has an additional ethical responsibility with regard to the prevention of injury by advising that appropriate equipment is worn by players, the environment is safe, and vulnerable individuals do not participate in an event when there is a risk of aggravating a primary injury or sustaining a second, invariably more serious injury – for example, advertising impediment and ancillary injurious materials such as photographic cameras!
>
> If a doctor recognises a pattern of events leading to injury, he has an ethical duty to draw it to the attention of the players, coaches and legislators, in the hope that this pattern can be broken and the injuries minimised.
>
> On occasion, the doctor may be faced with a situation where an injury has resulted from violence outside the rules of the game. This may occur as a result of careless or thoughtless play, but may be the result of deliberate cheating, recklessness or violence and, in these circumstances, the doctor has a duty both to treat the injured player and to protect other players from similar violence by informed liaison with the relevant official in the event club or sport and the individuals concerned [N.B. while preserving confidentiality through anonymity].

What Macleod has emphasized above is the abdication of any ethical guidelines in sport generally to protect the victims of violent criminally and civilly actionable foul play, in breach of the laws of any game, national and international, and also in breach of all civilized recognizable legal conduct. His thoughts in 1990 are now endorsed by the claim of the Canadian Center for Ethics in Sports, Professor Andrew Pipe in his feature *Reviving Ethics in Sports: Time for Physicians to Act* reproduced hereafter in Appendix III.

The law of the land does not stop at the touchline, or board or committee room. Since a grandstand collapsed at the traditional English Cheltenham race meeting in 1866, and a fatality occurred during a local Leicestershire football match in 1878, the English courts have charted an unbroken line of court actions to protect victims of violent foul play (see pp. 3, 50, *supra*).

Because hostility compounds ignorance in condemnation of this position, Macleod's conception is crucial for all concerned with the welfare within and outside sport in a civilized society; and his criteria for the 'environment is safe' was confirmed by Lord Justice Taylor's Hillsborough Report (see below). A valuable note in the *British Journal of Sports Medicine* from F. W. Smith at Woodend Hospital, Aberdeen (September 1998, Vol. 32, p. 198) exposes a lacuna in the Report's silence on a need for separate doctors for teams and crowds.

## FINAL REPORT: HILLSBOROUGH STADIUM DISASTER C.M. 962 BY HON LORD JUSTICE TAYLOR (1990)

*First Aid, Medical Facilities and Ambulances*

229. The scale of available medical facilities has been the subject of controversy. After Hillsborough, there were complaints of insufficient basic equipment such as stretchers. I repeat what I said in my Interim Report at paragraphs 298 and 299:

"298. It would be unreasonable to expect, at any sports stadium, medical facilities capable of dealing with a major disaster such as occurred. To have in advance at the ground, oxygen, resuscitators, stretchers, other equipment and medical staff sufficient to deal with over 100 casualties is not practicable.

299. What is required is a basic level of provision for first aid, for professional medical attention and for ambulance attendance, together with a system of co-ordination with the emergency services which will bring them to the scene swiftly in whatever numbers are required. What will amount to an appropriate basic provision for the future *eg* the equipment in a first aid room, requires expert evaluation and advice."

230. **The Scottish ambulance service has developed a "major incident equipment vehicle" designed and equipped to deal with up to 50 casualties. It is packed with 50 stretchers, blankets, and medical supplies and is in effect a travelling storehouse for such equipment. A**

vehicle of that type is deployed in addition to other ambulance attendance at matches with crowds over 25,000. This provision goes a long way towards meeting the criticism raised after Hillsborough and I recommend that it be adopted elsewhere.

231. I repeat the Interim Recommendations I made under this heading subject to two variations. First, it has been sensibly urged that it is unreasonable to require a medical practitioner to be present throughout a match where attendance is very small. At such a match it is suggested that to have a medical practitioner on call would be sufficient. I agree with this and recommend that the full-time presence of a doctor should not be required where there is no reasonable expectation of more than 2,000 spectators attending.

232. Secondly, some clubs have told me that they can secure private ambulance services more economically than those from the appropriate ambulance authority. They accordingly wish to have freedom to choose. I modify my Interim Recommendation in deference to this argument by requiring at least one fully equipped ambulance from, or approved by, the appropriate ambulance authority should be in attendance at all matches with an expected crowd of 5,000 or more.

**Table 11.1**    Disasters in football grounds outside the UK

| Venue | Year | Fatalities/injuries | Disaster/incident type |
|---|---|---|---|
| Ibague (Colombia) | 1961 | 11 dead, 15 injured | stand collapse |
| Santiago (Chile) | 1961 | 5 dead, 300 injured | crowd crush |
| Lima (Peru) | 1964 | 318 dead, 1000+ injured | riot |
| Istanbul (Turkey) | 1964 | 70 injured | fire |
| Kayseri (Turkey) | 1967 | 34 dead | riot |
| Buenos Aires (Argentina) | 1968 | 74 dead, 150 injured | disorder/stampede |
| Cairo (Egypt) | 1974 | 49 dead, 50 injured | crowd crush |
| Port-au-Prince (Haiti) | 1978 | 6 dead | disorder/police shooting |
| Piraeus (Greece) | 1981 | 21 dead, 54 injured | crush/stampede |
| San Luis (Brazil) | 1982 | 3 dead, 25 injured | riot/police shooting |
| Cali (Colombia) | 1982 | 24 dead, 250 injured | crushing/stampede |
| Algiers (Algeria) | 1982 | 10 dead, 500 injured | roof collapse |
| Moscow Spartak (Soviet Union) | 1982 | 69+ dead, 100+ injured | crowd crush |
| Heysel (Belgium) | 1985 | 38 dead, 400+ injured | disorder/wall collapse |
| Mexico City (Mexico) | 1985 | 10 dead, 100+ injured | crowd crush |
| Tripoli (Libya) | 1987 | 20 dead | unknown |

*(continued)*

**Table 11.1** (*cont.*)

| Venue | Year | Fatalities/injuries | Disaster/incident type |
|---|---|---|---|
| Katmandu (Nepal) | 1988 | 100 + dead, 500 injured | hailstorm/stampede |
| Lagos (Nigeria) | 1989 | 5 dead | crowd crush |
| Mogadishu (Somalia) | 1989 | 7 dead, 18 injured | riot |
| Orkney (South Africa) | 1991 | 42 dead, 50 injured | riot/stampede |
| Nairobi (Kenya) | 1991 | 1 dead, 24 injured | stampede |
| Rio de Janeiro (Brazil) | 1992 | 50 injured | fence collapse |
| Bastia (Corsica) | 1992 | 17 dead | temporary stand collapse |
| Free Town (Sierra Leone) | 1995 | 40 injured | gate collapse |
| Lusaka (Zambia) | 1996 | 9 dead, 52 injured | crowd crush |
| Guatemala | 1996 | 80 dead, 150 injured | crowd crush |

Reproduced from Frosdick, S. and Walley, L. (1997) *Sport and Safety Management*, Butterworth-Heinemann, Oxford, with permission.

**Table 11.2** Disasters and incidents involving United Kingdom stadia or supporters

| Venue | Year | Fatalities/injuries | Disaster/incident type |
|---|---|---|---|
| Valley Parade (Bradford)# | 1888 | 1 dead, 3 injured | railings collapse |
| Blackburn | 1896 | 5 injured | stand collapse |
| Ibrox (Glasgow) | 1902 | 26 dead, 550 injured | collapsed temporary stand |
| Brentford | 1907 | multiple injuries | fence collapse |
| Leicester | 1907 | multiple injuries | barrier collapse |
| Hillsborough (Sheffield) | 1914 | 70–80 injured | wall collapse |
| Charlton | 1923 | 24 injured | crowd crush |
| Wembley | 1923 | 1000 + injured | crowd crush |
| Burnley | 1924 | 1 dead | crowd crush |
| Manchester (City) | 1926 | unknown injuries | crowd crush |
| Huddersfield | 1932 | 100 injured | crowd crush |
| Huddersfield | 1937 | 4 injured | crowd crush |
| Watford | 1937 | unknown injuries | crowd crush |
| Fulham | 1938 | unknown injuries | crowd crush |
| Rochdale Athletic Ground# | 1939 | 1 dead, 17 injured | roof collapse |
| Burnden Park (Bolton) | 1946 | 33 dead, 400 injured | crowd crush |
| Shawfield (Clyde) | 1957 | 1 dead, 50 injured | barrier collapse |
| Ibrox (Glasgow) | 1961 | 2 dead, 50 injured | crowd crush on Stairway 13 |
| Oldham | 1962 | 15 injured | barrier collapse |
| Arsenal | 1963 | 100 injured | crushing |
| Port Vale | 1964 | 1 dead, 2 injured | fall/crushing |
| Roker Park (Sunderland) | 1964 | 80 + injured | crowd crush |
| Anfield (Liverpool) | 1966 | 31 injured | crowd crush |
| Leeds | 1967 | 32 injured | crowd crush |

(*continued*)

**Table 11.2** (*cont.*)

| Venue | Year | Fatalities/injuries | Disaster/incident type |
|---|---|---|---|
| Ibrox (Glasgow) | 1967 | 8 injured | crowd crush on Stairway 13 |
| Ibrox (Glasgow) | 1971 | 66 dead, 145 injured | crowd crush on Stairway 13 |
| Carlisle | 1971 | 5 injured | barrier collapse |
| Oxford | 1971 | 25 injured | wall collapse |
| Stoke | 1971 | 46 injured | crowd crush |
| Wolverhampton | 1972 | 80 injured | barrier collapse |
| Arsenal | 1972 | 42 injured | crowd crush |
| Lincoln | 1975 | 4 injured | wall collapse |
| Leyton Orient | 1978 | 30 injured | barrier/wall collapse |
| Middlesbrough | 1980 | 2 dead | gate collapse |
| Hillsborough (Sheffield) | 1981 | 38 injured | crowd crush |
| Walsall | 1984 | 20 injured | wall collapse |
| Bradford | 1985 | 54 dead | fire |
| Birmingham | 1985 | 1 dead, 20 injured | disorder/wall collapse |
| Heysel (Brussels) | 1985 | 38 dead, 400 + injured | disorder/wall collapse |
| Easter Road (Edinburgh) | 1987 | 150 injured | crowd crush |
| Hillsborough (Sheffield) | 1989 | 95 dead, 400 + injured | crowd crush |
| Middlesbrough | 1989 | 19 injured | crowd crush |

# Incident at rugby league ground.
Reproduced from Frosdick, S. and Walley, L. (1997) *Sport and Safety Management*, Butterworth-Heinemann, Oxford, with permission.

## THE RULE OF LAW IN SPORT
### Applied to injury examples proved or alleged to confirm Macleod's

additional ethical responsibility with regard to the prevention of injury by advising that ... the environment is safe (p. 122 *supra*)

**for Public Protection (A) Outside and (B) Inside Sports Grounds and Premises (reproduced and updated from Grayson, Edward: *Sport and the Law* (2nd edn, 1994) Butterworths: by kind permission of the publisher)**

### A: Public protection outside sports premises

**1922**
Golf ball played from the 13th tee parallel with Sandwich Road, Kent, much frequented by motor cars and taxi cabs, into which road golf ball was hit. Windscreen of passing taxi

**Decision**
Golf Club and player jointly liable for £450 damages and costs.
**Principle**
Tee and hole were *public nuisance* from the conditions and in the place

cab hit by ball and splintered glass, causing loss of driver's eye (*Castle v St Augustine's Links Ltd* (1922) 38 TLR 615).

where they were situated. No precedent for different facts: but slicing of ball into roadway not only a public danger but was the probable consequence from time to time of people driving from the tee.

**1949**
Supporters at Stamford Bridge, Chelsea, overflow onto neighbouring gardens after exclusion from Moscow Dynamo match in 1945 (*Munday v Metropolitan Police Receiver* [1949] 1 All ER 337).

**Decision**
Compensation against Receiver, Metropolitan Police.
**Principle**
Award under Riot Damages Act 1886 (still in force). Elements of riot proved under applicable law as at 1945, 1949.

**1950**
Noise from speedway track surrounding football ground disturbed occupiers of residential properties surrounding stadium (*Attorney General v Hastings Corporation* (1950) 94 Sol Jo 225).

**Decision**
Injunction against speedway noise obtained.
**Principle**
Nuisance to private interests overrode public interest in speedway competition.

**1951**
Cricket ball hit from Cheetham CC, Manchester to roadway on rare occasions (*Bolton v Stone* [1951] AC 850).

**Decision**
No liability.
**Principle**
No negligence or nuisance. Remote risk of injury not reasonably to be anticipated.

**1951**
Widow of deceased motor car race marshall sued organizers of race in Jersey and executors of the crashed car driver who also died (*O'Dowd v Frazer-Nash* [1951] WLR 173).

**Decision**
No liability.
**Principle**
Organizers had taken all reasonable precautions. No negligence by driver for brake failure.

**1961**
Footballs kicked out of field by young children (from green used frequently for recreational purposes) onto adjoining roadway. Motorcyclist thereby caused to swerve fatally (*Hilder v Associated Portland Cement Manufacturers* [1961] 1 WLR 1434).

**Decision**
Field owners liable for negligence.
**Principle**
Failure to take reasonable care from reasonably anticipated danger to road users.

**1968**
Pedestrian walking along narrow

**Decision**
Liability established for negligence.

## A: Public protection outside sports premises *(cont.)*

public lane injured on head by golf ball (*Lamond v Glasgow Corporation* (1968) SLT 291).

**Principle**
Although no previous history of any accident, 6000 shots a year played over fence should have created forecast of foreseeable happening.

### 1977
Cricket balls hit out of 70-year-old cricket club ground into adjoining gardens prevented occupants who had recently purchased house from using garden in summer (*Miller v Jackson* [1977] 1 QB 966).

**Decision**
Injunction discharged on appeal by club, but £400 agreed damages for nuisance.
**Principle**
On appeal, club guilty of nuisance and negligence; but Court of Appeal's discretion discharged injunction because public loss of cricket prevails over hardship from individual non-use of garden.

### 1981
Power-boat racing noise upset neighbour who built a house adjoining watersports lake (*Kennaway v Thompson* [1980] 3 All ER 329).

**Decision**
Damages award by trial judge of £15 000 discharged on appeal by householder, and replaced by modified injunction.
**Principle**
Courts do not approve the concept of wrongdoers purchasing potential to continue by merely paying for the injury. Injunction in modified but none the less effective terms to modify noise.

### 1994
Cricket balls hit into adjoining garden, protective fence required (*Lacey v Parker and Boyle* (for Jordans CC) [1994] 144 NLJ 785)

**Decision**
Injunction refused.
**Principle**
Plaintiff came to the nuisance, to which he objected only when cricket balls damaged his adjoining property.

## B: Public protection inside sports grounds and premises

### 1870
Collapsed Grandstand at Cheltenham Races (*Francis v Cockerell* [1870] 5 QB 501).

**Decision**
Judgment for spectator.
**Principle**
Negligently constructed stand for which promoter vicariously liable.

**1886**
Firework injury at (old) Crystal Palace (*Whitby v CJ Brock* (1886) 4 TLR 241).

**Decision**
Judgment for visitor.
**Principle**
Negligence proved.

**1896**
Collapsed grandstand at Blackburn Rovers (*Brown v Lewis* (1896) 12 TLR 455).

**Decision**
Judgment for spectator.
**Principle**
Negligent construction. Club committee members made personally liable.

**1932**
Polo player on pony ran through a hedge at Ranelagh injuring a spectator (*Piddington v Hastings* (1932) *Times*, 12 March p. 4).

**Decision**
Judgment for owners of premises.
**Principle**
No failure by premises owners to use reasonable care.

**1932**
Motor race track. Contact of wheels at 100 mph between two Talbot racing cars caused one apparently to leave the track and go over rails at side of track (*Hall v Brooklands Auto-Racing Club* [1933] 1 KB 205).

**Decision**
Judgment for owners of premises and competitors.
**Principle**
No evidence per Court of Appeal that owners or competitors had failed to take reasonable care.

**1949**
Ice hockey players stepped out of or broke off from hockey game to fight, injuring spectator with stick (*Payne and Payne v Maple Leaf* (1949) 1 DLR 369 (Canada)).

**Decision**
Players liable.
**Principle**
No consent to breach of rules.

**1951**
Ice hockey puck hit 6-year-old rinkside spectator (*Murray v Haringay Arena* [1951] 2 KB 529.

**Decision**
Judgment for owners.
**Principle**
No lack of safety.

**1962**
Photographer at horse show injured by winning horse (*Wooldridge v Sumner* [1963] 2 QB 43).

**Decision**
Judgment for organizers and competitor.
**Principle**
No lack of safety.

**1971**
Spectators injured at motor-cycle scramble meeting (*Wilkes v Cheltenham Home Guard Motor Cycle and Light Car Club* [1971] 3 All ER 369, CA).

**Decision**
No liability.
**Principle**
Almost inexplicable accident. Competitors and organizers exonerated from negligence. Competitor entitled to strain to win if not foolhardy.

## B. Public protection inside sports ground and premises (*cont.*)

**1974**

Spectators at 1971 Ibrox disaster (*Dougan v Rangers Football Club* (1974) *Daily Telegraph*, 24 October p. 19).

**Decision**

Judgment for representatives of deceased victims. Glasgow Rangers liable.

**Principle**

Failed to exercise sufficient care to spectators in egress and handrails prior to 1975 Act.

**1976**

Discus hurled from practice net on athletics ground ricocheted from guy-rope and hit spectator standing well behind the net (*Wilkins v Smith* (1976) 73 LS Gaz 839).

**Decision**

Judgment for owners.

**Principle**

Duty fulfilled by keeping spectators out of the area of foreseeable deflection.

**1987**

Bradford City Fire disaster (*Fletcher and Fletcher; Britton v Bradford City Association Football Club and others* (1987) *Times, Daily Telegraph*, 24 February).

**Decision**

Judgment for victims.

**Principle**

Negligence by club and local Fire Authority.

**1987**

Sheffield United Special Police Services (*Harris v Sheffield United Football Club Limited* [1987] 2 All ER 838).

**Decision**

£51 699.54 liability of club to South Yorkshire Police Authority.

**Principle**

Special police services for soccer crowd problems chargeable for beyond normal public duty to maintain law and order.

**1991**

Occupier football club liable to injured Police when visiting Bristol City fans threw missiles from dilapidated premises (*Cunningham v Reading FC Ltd* (1991) *Times*, 20 March).

**Decision**

Judgment for injured Police Officers from hooligans on Football Club premises.

**Principle**

Crowd law negligence and Occupiers Act 1957, s 2 (1), (2) established because of prior knowledge of club about a violent element among particular visiting supporters.

**1991**

Insufficient ties of 'love and affection' or physical closeness to victims of stadium disaster at the time of events (*Alcock v Chief Constable of*

**Decision**

Judgment for Defendant against Hillsborough claimants.

**Principle**

Only those present in stadium and

*South Yorkshire Police* [1991] 4 All ER 907).

**1993**
Injuries resulting from open hole or underlying void in racetrack on occasion of 1989 St Leger autumn meeting (*Cook, Cochrane, Hampson v Doncaster Borough Council* (1993) *Sporting Life*, 16 July).

**1996**
Footballer in losing control of ball collided with plaintiff on crowd control duty watching spectators, and propelled her into barrier, causing injury (*Gillon v Chief Constable of Strathclyde Police and Anor* (1996) *Times*, 22 November).

not those watching on television qualified to claim disaster damages.

**Decision**
Judgment for jockeys and racehorse owner.
**Principle**
Defendant corporation controlling owners of the racetrack surface liable for unsatisfactory conditions creating negligence liability.

**Decision**
Judgment for Defendant against woman police sergeant plaintiff.
**Principle**
Minimal foreseeable risk of injury.

Chapter 12

# Conclusion: Evidence, ethics, injuries and the law in sport and sports medicine

The saga of *Ethics, Injuries and the Law in Sports Medicine* has one connecting thread linking all these disparate elements under the heading of evidence. The establishment of *facts*, whether for a clinical diagnosis or legal liability, is universally recognized.

## MEDICAL FACTS AND ADMISSIBLE LEGAL EVIDENCE FOR SPORTING INJURIES

For sports medical and paramedical practitioners, two vivid sources explain the position clearly and simply. One of the century's leading physicians in the first half of this century, Lord Horder, is recalled in a memoir by his son, Mervyn Horder (*The Little Genius*, 1966) who relates how his father built his diagnostic reputation on his:

> pre-occupation with the post-mortem room ... and an examination of the body after death was, as it sometimes still is, the only way to arrive at the truth about a particular case, to confirm or upset a diagnosis, and to push forward the frontiers of knowledge in general. There is no arguing with the corpse on the slab.

The corollary to this appears in the current (13th edn) *Glaister's Medical Jurisprudence and Toxicology* (Glaister, 1973). Written initially by successive holders of the Regius Chair of Forensic Medicine in the University of Glasgow, John Glaister Snr, and his son John Glaister Jnr, the conclusions to the chapter entitled 'The medico-legal aspects of wounds' advise (at p. 256):

> ... the examiner should direct his attention to the reconstruction of the cause of the injuries. He should first decide the instrument, then the degree of violence, the possibility of accident, the direction of the wound, and the relative position of the parties.

These two definitive sources from separate periods of time lead in naturally to the landmark publications in the *British Medical*

*Journal* for December 1978 from J. P. R. Williams and Professor John Davies and Terry Gibson (1978), and a year later when P. N. Sperryn (1979) in the paper to the British Association of Sports Medicine symposium published in the *British Journal of Sports Medicine*, vol 14, nos 2&3 August 1980, pp. 84–9, reaffirmed:

> It has recently become evident that deliberate foul play in certain sports is directly responsible for many sports injuries. It could be argued that the medical profession, on becoming aware of trends in the style of play in sport, should be among the first to initiate the political changes which should lead to elimination of dangerous unfair play.

Thus, Donald Macleod's guidelines confirm:

> If a doctor recognises a pattern of events leading to injury, he has an ethical duty to draw it to the attention of the players, coaches and legislators, in the hope that this pattern can be broken and the injuries minimised.

## MEDICO-LEGAL FACTS AND ADMISSIBLE EVIDENCE IN THE LAW FOR SPORTING INJURIES

Comparable to the Horder–Glaister guidelines for factual foundations for clinical diagnosis is a crucial but oft-forgotten *Report of the Committee on Legal Education* (Cmnd 4595). It was commissioned by Lord Gardiner, Lord Chancellor in 1967, and completed for his successor, Lord Hailsham of St Marylebone in 1971, under the chairmanship of Mr Justice (later Lord Justice) Ormrod. It explained the realities underlying this aspect of the administration of justice, in para 91 at p. 38, thus (with my own emphasis):

> The raw material of every *practising lawyer* is facts, and a great deal of his time will be spent, whether he is a judge or a barrister or a solicitor, *in finding the facts*. The law cannot be properly applied until they are ascertained. If the facts are wrong, the advice of the most learned lawyer will be, at best, worthless – and may be dangerous. Facts, therefore are of crucial importance to the practising lawyer at all levels, and his ability to *handle* facts is among his most essential skills. The *handling* of facts has many aspects. The practitioner must first *obtain* the client's instructions and the surrounding facts, and then *investigate* and *scrutinise* them for accuracy. Analysis of all the available data, to separate the *relevant* from the irrelevant and to perceive the relation between one set of facts and another and so to check reliability or expose errors, is an essential process in every case. In every case, also, he must *synthesise* his facts in order to present them lucidly and cogently, whether as an advocate, or as a pleader, or as a draftsman, or negotiator, or even as a letter writer. All stages of

these processes will of course be controlled and informed by his knowledge of the relevant law, without which the exercise would be futile.

The emphasis on italicized words here is made deliberately. To *find, obtain, handle, investigate, scrutinize* and *synthesize* relevant *facts* is a process in which both branches of practising lawyers depend upon other people for providing the facts.

Every practitioner familiar with sports-related injuries will have his or her own examples, where the two medico-legal disciplines merge to produce a positive result. For this author, a classic illustration occurred before the Criminal Injuries Compensation Board in 1991.

A third XV rugby player lost an eye in a line-out. He was unable to identify the offender. Two of his colleagues were able to do so, but without the required degree of certainly (beyond reasonable doubt) to persuade the police to charge; and, in any event, the first base filter process at the CICB did not consider that criminality could be established.

This double denial of redress was rebutted by a perfect mixture of medical and legal evidence. Specialist ophthalmic surgical evidence established both that only a sharp instrument (such as a thumb and/ or knuckle) was consistent with the eye injury, and the requisite criminal evidentiary elements of deliberation and/or recklessness (see *R v Bradshaw* (1878) 14 Cox CC 83), and a serving Metropolitan Police Chief Superintendent George Crawford, who was also a rugby union referee of international standards, confirmed in evidence that a breach of Laws of the Game spilled over into a breach of sections 18 or 20 of the Offences Against the Person Act, 1861.

By contrast, three examples from comparatively recent cases illustrate the problems inherent in the selection and applicability of the appropriate evidence from specialist sources which is often required for establishing or rejecting liability for sporting injuries:

1   *Smoldon v Whitworth and Nolan* (1997) (*Times*, 19 April; *Times*, 18 December, 1996). Curtis J and the Court of Appeal respectively utilized the *defendant witness* referee's/specialist evidence in favour of the *plaintiff* of the Defendant's negligent scrum laws of the game.

2   *Fowles v Bedfordshire County Council* (1995) (PIQR P380). A gymnast who slipped on a mat claimed damages, established a one-third liability against the defendant council, but with a two-thirds contributory negligence reduction found against himself per, *inter alia*, Millett LJ in the Court of Appeal at

p. 388 who recorded how the plaintiff's expert witnesses were 'stunned' by his 'utter foolishness'.

3  *Murray v Haringay Arena* [1951] 2 KB, 529. This relatively old but nonetheless oft-cited leading case, to support the proposition that there is no obligation to guard against unusual dangers at sports venues, rejected a six year-old's appeal from a claim for an eye injury at an ice-rink, Singleton LJ at pp. 531–2 said:

> The evidence given on the hearing was meagre. There was no evidence from anyone connected with the management; no evidence to show how long the rink had been in existence: no evidence to show the number of persons who normally attended matches; and no evidence to show whether there had been any other accidents there. In a sense this appears to be unsatisfactory, and yet it would seem that there are ways in which the plaintiffs might have obtained information on these matters.

While the civil and criminal compensation damages awards and criminal prosecutions continue to unfold for sport-related issues, financial rewards for talent increase concurrently. To guide such talents many services are required from professionals such as accountants and lawyers. Furthermore, solicitor members of the legal profession have been authorized by the Law Society in England to act as agents, for FIFA and the FA both in legal and commercial areas. Accordingly, an at-present unresolved ethical crisis exists for the legal and accountancy professions in to what extent are they obliged to warn their clients ethically how breaches of playing law required application of Macleod's guidelines.

Finally, as a warning from the past, with a built-in caution for the present and future, sports medical practitioners at all levels should bear in mind two precedents midway through the present century which are rarely recalled but merit consideration for their hidden meaning today.

*Clarke v Adams* 1950 (Sol Jnl) was a decision by Slade J for injury suffered by a Plaintiff who had been treated by the defendant physiotherapist for a fibrotic condition of his left heel. In the process of short-wave diathermy treatment the Plaintiff suffered burning which was so bad that his left leg had to be amputated below the knee. The physiotherapist had given the following warning to the patient in accordance with the correct professional procedure confirmed by the expert testimony of the Chief Examiner for the Chartered Society of Physiotherapy:

> When I turn on the machine I want you to experience a comfortable warmth and nothing more, if you do I want you to tell me.

The apparatus was not defective but inherently dangerous because burns caused by it could lead to serious consequences. Slade J held that the warning given was insufficiently clear to create a warning of danger, notwithstanding the testimony of correct practice, and thereby amounted to negligent conduct. The case was decided seven years after *Bolam*, but on the evidence available in the reported sources the result turned upon the adjudged inadequacy of the warning of danger. Whether this decision would be reconsidered if ever argued in a subsequent case is a matter reflecting a wider issue. Precision of language and communication and comprehension between practitioner and patient are as crucial in practice as awareness of correct ethical and legal guidelines in sport and the wider society.

One other experience from 1950 is as convenient a note as any on which to end these pages. For it poses a question which may be unanswerable yet should not be ignored in the current climate of assessing performance enhancement substances. Arsenal Football Club, the current FA Cup and Premier League double champions, triumphed in the 1950 FA Cup Final by a 2–0 victory against Liverpool. One of its heroes was the late Denis Compton CBE, already identified in these pages as a true Corinthian in the spirit of fair play. In both his biography by Tim Heald and an interview with Norman Giller, each published before he died on St George's Day 1997, the story is told of his half-time tonic from another Arsenal hero from the inter-war years before 1939, Alex James. 'Get this down you', whispered James, handing Compton a small glass of liquid. He looked at it, smelt it and pulled a face. It was brandy. As Compton said to Norman Giller:

> I decided that Alex had been around in the game long enough to know what he was doing, and so I drank the brandy in one go. Whether it was psychological or what I don't know, but it certainly put the snap back in my game in the second half and I felt quite pleased with my contribution to our 2–0 victory.

This cheerful admission can justifiably be the starting point for all concerned with the Danish Medical Association's paper to be considered at the WMA meeting at Ottawa in October 1998 and the IOC conference at Lausanne in February 1999 for evaluating what is a performance enhancing substance, for all participants in sport at any level, from the grassroots to the public arena.

Thus, an appropriate note on which to end this whole text, is to recall what as long ago as 1979 Sir Roger Bannister (the first four-minute mile record-holder, neurologist and later Master of Pembroke College, Oxford), wrote in his foreword to *Fair Play: Ethics in Sport and Education* (McIntosh (1979)):

It is an increasingly popular notion among many young people that we can throw off ethical and moral principles in more and more spheres of life ... The fact of the matter is that we are faced with moral choices many times a day and if we do not notice them it must be that our intelligence or sensitivity is becoming blunted. Sport, which occupies the professional time of a few and the spare time of many, is a fit study for ethics.

Those ethics merged with Bannister's dual careers as athlete and doctor after he broke the four-minute mile barrier in 1954 as a medical student on Oxford University's Iffley Road running track, almost symbolically a year after BASM's foundation in 1953. They echoed a long tradition of United Kingdom sporting medical practitioners, illustrated vividly from the world's two most popular team games while these pages approached conclusion in 1998.

Cricket's domain celebrated the 150th birthday anniversary of its first international cult hero, Dr W. G. Grace. Fifteen years earlier Robert A. Kyle MD and Marc A. Shampo PhD, in the *Journal of the American Medical Association* (3 June 1983, vol. 249, no. 21, p. 2912 recorded:

> William Gilbert Grace, a physician [a local Bristol GP] is remembered as an outstanding cricketer rather than by any contribution to medicine or science.

Yet the worldwide commemoration of his birth evidenced the enduring legacy of his cricketing greatness. Towards the end of Grace's era in the 1890s, an earlier Oxford University medical student before Bannister's period began his progression towards appointments as physician to two Kings of England (George V and George VI), and Regius Professor of Medicine at Oxford University, among countless other honours as a distinguished clinician and neurologist. The late Sir Edward Farquhar Buzzard, Bart, began his *Who's Who* entry with membership of Oxford University Association Football XIs of 1892–4; the Old Carthusian FA Amateur Cup winning XIs of 1895 and 1897 and the London Senior Cup Finals of 1895, 1896 and 1897. In 1998 the University Association Football Club's history under the authorship of Colin Weir records his Presidency of it until he died in 1945. His immortal Oxford and Corinthian contemporary C. B. Fry wrote of him in *Life Worth Living* (1939) he 'was a strong player at left-half-back. I hope he is as good a Regius Professor as he was a footballer'. Indeed, he was; and the present international standing of the Oxford University Medical Faculty and Nuffield Trust are a monument to his personal development of them. On his death, the *Lancet* obituary notice of 29 December, 1945 (vol. 3, p. 864) recorded his advice, with an aptness for today:

The doctor in a hurry is a menace to his patient. The most important difference between the good and indifferent clinician is the amount of time he pays to the story of the patient.

It is an appropriate note on which to end this story, too.

# References

Asken, M. *Dying to Win* (cited in Canadian Government's *Commission of Inquiry into the Use of Drugs and Banned Practices Intended to Increase Athletic Performance*. Mr Justice Dubin).

Ayer, A. J. (1972–73) *Philosophy and Science*, First Gifford Lecture, St Andrews University.

Bannister, R. (1979) Foreword to P. McIntosh, *Fair Play: Ethics in Sport and Education*, Heinemann Educational.

Beckett, A. H. (1981) The problems of drugs in sport. In: *Dictionary of Medical Ethics* (2nd edn).

Berry, R. C. and Wong, G. M. (1993) *Law and Business of the Sports Industries*, Westport.

Betts, J. C. (1990) Scuba-diving and its medical problems: the role of the doctor. In: *Medicine, Sport and the Law* (S. D. W. Payne, ed.), pp. 295–6, Blackwell Scientific Publications.

Bianco, E. and Walker, E. J. (1994) Legal aspects of sport medicine. In: *Sports Medicine for the Primary Care Physician* (2nd edn), (R. B. Birrer, ed.), p. 3, CRC Press.

Birrer, R. B. (ed.) (1994) *Sports Medicine for the Primary Care Physician* (2nd edn), CRC Press.

BMA (1993) *Medical Ethics Today: Its Practice and Philosophy*, Medical Ethics Committee Working Party, BMJ Publishing Group.

BMA (1995) *ABC of Sports Medicine* (G. McLatchie *et al*, eds), BMJ Publishing Group.

BMA Board of Science and Education (1996) *Sport and Exercise Medicine: Policy and Provision*, BMJ Publishing Group.

Bottomley, M. (1990) Athletes at an overseas venue: the role of the team doctor. In: *Medicine, Sport and the Law* (S. D. W. Payne, ed.), Blackwell Scientific Publications.

*Bulletin of Medical Ethics* (1998), May.

Carey, G., Archbishop of Canterbury (1996) 5 July, *Moral and Spiritual Wellbeing*, House of Lords. *Hansard* Vol. 573.

*Commission of Enquiry into the Use of Drugs and Banned Practices Intended to Increase Athletic Performance* (1990) Canadian Government.

Comyn, J. (1993) *Watching Brief, Further Memoirs of an Irishman in England*, The Round Hall Press.

Crane, J. (1990) Association football: the team doctor. In: *Medicine, Sport and the Law* (S. D. W. Payne, ed.), Blackwell Scientific Publications.

Davies, J. E. and Gibson, T. (1978) Injuries in rugby union football. *Br. Med. J.*, p. 1759.

D'Israeli, B. (1845) *Sybil: or The Two Nations*, Henry Colburn.

Doggart, H. (1994) The Corinthian Ideal, Appendix 1, *Sport and the Law* (2nd edn), Butterworths.

Donohue, T. and Johnson, N. (1986) *Foul Play: Drug Abuse in Sports*, Blackwell Scientific Publications.

Drake, M. (1997) *Guilty of Wanting to Win: Penal Liability in Sports Activity*, Italian Olympic Committee.

Dubin, C. L. (1990) *Commission of Inquiry into the Use of Drugs and Banned Practices Intended to Increase Athletic Performance*, Canadian Government.

Farber, J. (1980) *A Code of Ethics for Sports Medicine*, World Medical Association.

Franck, A. and Olagnier, H. (1996) Consentiment et dependence pour l'adolescent sportif de haut-niveau. *Medecine et Hygiene*, **54**, 1393–6.

Gallup, E. M. (1995) *Law and the Team Physician*, Human Kinetics.

Garraway, M., McLeod, D. and Sharpe, J. C. M. (1991) Rugby injuries devised for case registers, *Br. Med. J.*, **303**, 1082–3.

General Medical Council (1993) *Tomorrow's Doctors*.

Glaister, J. Sr and Jr (1973) *Glaister's Medical Jurisprudence and Toxicology* (13th edn), Churchill Livingstone.

Grant, E. (1985) *The Bitter Pill: How Safe is the 'Perfect Contraceptive'?*, Corgi Books.

Grayson, E. (1992) *Sports Medicine Distant Learning Course for Doctors*, Module 7, pp. 43–4, University of Bath.

Grayson, E. (1994) *Sport and the Law* (2nd edn), Butterworths.

Grayson, E. (1996) *Corinthians and Cricketers: and Towards a New Sporting Era*, Yore Publications.

Greenberg, M. J. (1996) Unpublished manuscript.

Greenway, P. and Greenway, M. (1997) General practitioner knowledge of prohibited substances in sport, *Br. J. Sports Med.*, **31**, 129–31.

Grisogono, V. (1994) *Children and Sport: Fitness, Injuries and Diet*, John Murray.

Hailsham, Lord (1990) *A Sparrow's Flight*, Collins.

Hall, M. R. P., MacLennan, W. J. and Lye, M. D. (1993) *Medical Care for the Elderly*, Wiley.

Harding, T. (1996) The ethical issues and potential abuses of adolescents' participation in high-level sport, *Lancet*, **348**, 400.

Harries, M., Williams, C., Standish, W. and Michali, L. (eds) (1994) *Oxford Textbook of Sports Medicine*, Oxford University Press.

Henderson, J. M. (1998) In: *Sports Pharmacology. Clinics in Sports Medicine*, W. B. Saunders.

Hoddle, G. with Davies, D. (1998) *My 1998 World Cup Story*, André Deutsch Classics.

Hollman, W. (1988) The definition and scope of sports medicine. In: *The Olympic Book of Sports Medicine* (A. Dirix, H. G. Knutten and K. Tittel, eds), Blackwell Scientific Publications.

Horder, T. M. (1966) *The Little Genius*, Duckworth.

International Code of Medical Ethics, Declaration of Geneva, WMA.

International Labour Office (1998) *Professional Sports Encyclopaedia of Occupational Health*, vol. 3.

Italian National Olympic Committee (1997) *Guilty of Wanting to Win*.

Jackson, R. M. and Powell, J. L. (1997) *Professional Negligence*, Sweet & Maxwell.

Johnson, R. J. and Lombardo, J. (eds) (1998) *Current Review of Sports Medicine* (2nd edn), Butterworth-Heinemann.

Johnston, W. (1983) *On the Wing*, Barker.

Jones, M. A. (1996) *Medical Negligence* (2nd edn), Sweet & Maxwell.

Kennedy, I. and Grubb, A. (1994) *Medical Law: Text with Materials* (2nd edn), Butterworths.

Kennedy, I. and Grubb, A. (eds) (1998) *Principles of Medical Law*, Oxford University Press.

Klenerman, L. (1994) Musculoskeletal injuries in child athletics. In: *ABC of Sports Medicine* (G. McLatchie *et al*, eds), BMJ Publishing Group.

Knill-Jones, R. (1997) Sports injury clinics, *Br. J. Sports Med.*, **31**, 95–6.

Kyle, R. A. and Shampo, M. A. (1983) *Journal of the American Medical Association*, **249**, 21, 2912.

McCauley, D. (1997) Editorial. *Br. J. Sports Med.*, June.

McIntosh, P. (1979) *Fair Play: Ethics in Sport and Education*, Heinemann Educational.

Macleod, D. (1990) The doctor's contribution to safety in sport. In: *Medicine Sport and the Law* (S. D. W. Payne, ed.), Blackwell Scientific Publications.

Macleod, D. (1995) Team medical care. In: *ABC of Sports Medicine* (G. McLatchie *et al*, eds), BMJ Publishing Group.

Macleod, D. (1996) Editorial. *Br. J. Sports Med.*

Magnusson, R. S. and Opie, H. (1990) HIV and hepatitis in sport. A legal framework for resolving hard cases. *Monash University Law Review* (Editorial).

Mant, A. K. (1986). *Br. Med. J.*, 29 November.

Mason, J. K. and McCall-Smith, R. A. (1981) *Law and Medical Ethics* (1st edn), Butterworths.

Mason, J. K. and McCall-Smith, R. A. (1991) *Law and Medical Ethics* (3rd edn), Butterworths.

Mason, J. K. and McCall-Smith, R. A. (1994) *Law and Medical Ethics* (4th edn), Butterworths.

Mellion, M. B. and Walsh, W. M. (1990) The team physician. In: *The Team Physician's Handbook* (M. B. Mellion *et al*, eds), Mosby.

Morgan, Cliff (1998) *Sport on Four*, BBC.

Peterson, L. and Reström, P. (1983) *Sports Injuries: Their Prevention and Treatment*, Swedish Sports Federation.

Pipe, A. (1998) Reviving ethics in sports: time for physicians to act, *Physician Sports Med.*, **26** (6).

Powers, M. J. and Harris, N. H. (1994) *Medical Negligence* (2nd edn), Butterworths.

Report of Committee on Legal Education (1971) Cmnd 4595.

Roberts, W. O. (1998) Keeping sport safe: physicians should take the lead, *Physician Sports Med.*, **26** (5).

Ryan, J. L. (1996) *Little Girls in Pretty Boxes*, Warner Books.

Scott, J. (1989) *Caught in Court*, Deutsch.

Scottish Royal Colleges Board for Sports Medicine (1989).

Silver, J. R. and Stewart, D. (1994) The prevention of spinal injuries in rugby football, *J. Int. Soc. Paraplegia*, **32** (7), 442.

Sperryn, P. N. (1979) Paper to the British Association of Sports Medicine Symposium, *Br. J. Sports Med.*, **14**, 84–9.

*Sports Illustrated* (1994) 40th Anniversary 1954–1994.

Warnock, M. (1998) *An Intelligent Person's Guide to Ethics*, Duckworth.

Weiler, P. C. and Roberts, G. R. (1998) *Sports and the Law: Texts, Cases, Problems* (2nd edn), West Group.

Weir, C. (1998) *History of Oxford University Association Football Club 1872–1998*, Yore Publications.

Wilkinson, N. (1990) The pill that can kill sports (cited in Dubin Report).

Williams, A., Evans, R. and Shirley, P. (1989) *Imaging of Sports Injuries*, Ballière Tindall.

Williams, J. P. R. and McKibbin (1978) Cervical spine injuries in rugby football, *Br. Med. J.*, 1747.

Williams, M. *Drugs and Athletic Performance*.

Williams, R. (1997) On the million dollar girls and the tightrope they walk on the demanding tennis circuit. *London Evening Standard*, 27 June.

Wooldridge, I. (1994) *Sport on Four*, BBC.

Young, A. (1995) *Medicine for Sport for Medicine*, Institute of Sports Medicine Lecture.

Appendix I

# A code of ethics for sports medicine*

by Dr J. Farber, Chairman of the Committee on Medical Ethics.
Reproduced with permission from the *Journal of the World Medical
Association.*

## PREAMBLE

It would be helpful to start by pointing out the distinction between
sport as a recreation, and competitive sport as practised by
professionals, for the doctor specializing in sports medicine has a
fundamentally different role according to which of these his patient
engages in.

For recreational sport, the doctor has first and foremost to be on
the lookout for contraindications to the desired sporting activity as
much before as during the event.

The doctor must always be in a position to advise against
participation in a sport which, whether through age or illness, has
become harmful to his patient. The work of this doctor will bring
him up against various obstacles, not least of which is the argument
whether sporting activities really do have a beneficial effect on health.

While nobody denies the mental and physical satisfaction as well
as the sense of well-being which usually accompany participation in
sports, by the same token neither can anybody maintain that in
practice this lowers risk of illness – the very opposite in fact.

The role of the doctor in this type of activity remains that of
adviser, just as it is for all the other activities in which people take
part.

In the case of *competitive* sport, here the doctor plays a more
active, even more aggressive role.

The patients he tends are in effect professionals. Their activity
differs from that of other occupations in several respects: their
career is shorter; their income is derived not from a continuous

* A working paper for consideration at the October 1980 Council Session, Munich.
Translated from the original French and not yet seen by the author.

routine but from a certain number of short bursts of effort, short events according to the outcome of which they have lost everything or gained everything. Their success depends entirely on pulling off a series of outstanding performances.

These professionals are besides subjected to physical strains theoretically beyond the bounds of endurance for the average person.

Finally, the very high level of international competition makes it impossible to shine without holding the winning cards.

It is well known that since the era of the Olympic Games of Ancient Greece, sportsmen have undergone special training regimes, in short put themselves in condition in order to take part in events. Similarly at all times sportsmen have used means urged on them by their trainers which, when discovered, led to disqualification. Nowadays those in competitive sports are put through the mill by physicians who subject competitors to modern pharmacological drug-detection tests. However, there is a difference between sending a sportsman to a high-altitude locality for some weeks to increase his erythrocyte count, and reinfusing his own previously withdrawn blood, as occurred in the case of the winner of the 5000 metres track event at Montreal.

What distinction should one draw between body-building by muscular exercise and that acquired by injection of anabolic agents?

It is well known that those taking part in rifle matches use tranquillizers and beta-blockers, and that champion weight-lifters can only engage in their arduous competitions at the cost of anaesthetic injections into the knee ligaments.

It therefore strikes us as essential that we face up to the reality of medical practices in competitive sports rather than deplore them or try vainly to forbid them.

## GENERAL PRINCIPLES

*Amateur sports*

The patient who consults a doctor over his fitness for sport has a right to the same ethical and scientific consideration from this doctor as in any other consultation. The doctor will give his totally objective opinion. He will only be free to communicate to third parties his bare conclusions as to the candidate's fitness or otherwise for sports.

The doctor has the duty, when he thinks indicated, to recommend medical supervision at sports proceedings and to submit his own competence to periodical review.

The doctor will pay special attention to the supervision of children and adolescents engaging in sports.

The doctor will forbid the use of any artificial means of improving performance and will look for evidence thereof at the time of the competition.

### Competitive professional sports

It is incumbent upon the doctor to keep the professional sportsman constantly informed of the consequences for health of the matches in which he takes part and of the means both natural and artificial which he may use to enhance his performance.

The doctor will avoid use of these means when they could be harmful to the sportsman's future and especially when they concern children and adolescents, in whom the use of such means should be vigorously proscribed.

The doctor will oppose the use by the sportsman of artificial methods the efficacity and relative harmlessness of which have not been scientifically demonstrated.

In carrying out physical and pharmacodynamic procedures the doctor will not enter into any exclusive contract with the sportsman or group of sportsmen.

If the regular medical attendant so requests, the sports doctor will pass on to him all the relevant information about the treatments he has given their common patient. The sports doctor will take part in scientific meetings at which techniques for the improvement of performance will be discussed.

These discussions will be published in a form accessible to all doctors.

In so far as the rules enacted by sports associations or the laws of the land and regulations appertaining to this matter expressly forbid it, the doctor will refrain from giving treatments intended to enhance performance to those professional athletes who may request them.

Similarly the doctor will refrain from giving such treatments without the sportsman's knowledge.

When there is some contraindication to engaging in a sport as a professional the doctor will so inform the sportsman concerned and, together with his regular doctor, will take all necessary steps to deter the athlete from such injurious exertions.

Like every other doctor the sports doctor, in his dealings with sports professionals, is bound to secrecy in regard to third parties.

Appendix II

# World Medical Association declaration on principles of health care for sports medicine

The World Medical Association (WMA) is an independent confederation of professional medical associations from approximately 70 different countries. The organization is an apolitical body which provides a forum for its member associations to communicate with each other, and to achieve consensus on the highest possible standards of medical ethics and professional competence. Since the establishment of the WMA in 1947, this organization has become an authoritative voice, offering physicians guidance through its Declarations and Statements. These also help to guide national medical associations, governments and international organizations throughout the world.

The principles of health care as practised in sports medicine have been an important issue to physicians worldwide. This was confirmed by the 34th WMA General Assembly in 1981 held in Lisbon, Portugal. Here the WMA adopted a Declaration to act as a guideline to physicians treating athletes. It is important to realize the significance of a Declaration: first a member country or countries propose a certain declaration on a relevant issue. This proposal is critically assessed by the WMA members, after which the issue is debated at one of the Standing Committees, then the WMA Council and eventually the full Assembly. A Declaration passed is therefore truly a representative global opinion on a certain matter.

Because declarations need revision in the light of new knowledge, the WMA Declaration on the Principles of Health Care for Sports Medicine has been amended on two occasions:

- By the 39th WMA General Assembly in Madrid, Spain (October 1987)
- By the 45th WMA General Assembly in Budapest, Hungary (October 1993)

In the light of the world-wide attention on 'doping and sport', the

WMA will again look at this declaration when the organization's members meet in Ottawa, Canada during October 1998, to make sure that the present guidelines are comprehensive and appropriate enough.

## WORLD MEDICAL ASSOCIATION DECLARATION ON PRINCIPLES OF HEALTH CARE FOR SPORTS MEDICINE

Adopted by the 34th World Medical Assembly, Lisbon, Portugal, September/October 1981; and amended by the 39th World Medical Assembly, Madrid, Spain, October 1987; and the 45th World Medical Assembly, Budapest, Hungary, October 1993.

The WMA has drafted and recommends the following ethical guidelines for physicians in order to meet the needs of the sportsmen or athletes and the special circumstances in which the medical care and health guidance is given. Consequently,

1   The physician who cares for sportsmen or athletes has an ethical responsibility to recognize the special physical and mental demands placed upon them by their performance in sports activities.

2   When the sports participant is a child or an adolescent, the physician must give first consideration to the participant's growth and stage of development.

   2.1   The physician must ensure that the child's state of growth and development, as well as his or her general condition of health can absorb the rigours of the training and competition without jeopardizing the normal physical or mental development of the child or adolescent.

   2.2   The physician must oppose any sports or athletic activity that is not appropriate to the child's stage of growth and development or general condition of health. The physician must act in the best interest of the health of the child or adolescent, without regard to any other interest or pressure from any other source.

3   When the sports participant is a professional sportsman or athlete and derives livelihood from that activity, the physician should pay due regard to the occupational medical aspects involved.

4   The physician should oppose the use of any method which is not in accordance with professional ethics, or which might be harmful to the sportsman or athlete using it, especially:

   4.1   Procedures which artificially modify blood constituents or biochemistry.

   4.2   The use of drugs or other substances whatever their nature and route of administration, including central-nervous-system stimulants or depressants and procedures which artificially modify reflexes.

4.3 Induced alterations of will or general mental outlook.

4.4 Procedures to mask pain or other protective symptoms if used to enable the sportsman or athlete to take part in events when lesions or signs are present which make his participation inadvisable.

4.5 Measures which artificially change features appropriate to age and sex.

4.6 Training and taking part in events when to do so would not be compatible with preservation of the individual's fitness, health or safety.

4.7 Measures aimed at an unnatural increase or maintenance of performance during competition. Doping to improve an athlete's performance is unethical.

5  The physician should inform the sportsman or athlete, those responsible for him, and other interested parties, of the consequences of the procedures he is opposing, guard against their use, enlist the support of other physicians and other organizations with the same aim, protect the sportsman or athlete against any pressures which might induce him to use these methods and help with supervision against these procedures.

6  The sports physician has the duty to give his objective opinion on the sportsmen or athletes' fitness or unfitness clearly and precisely, leaving no doubt as to his conclusions.

7  In competitive sports or professional sports events, it is the physician's duty to decide whether the sportsman or athlete can remain on the field or return to the game. This decision cannot be delegated to other persons. In the physician's absence these individuals must adhere strictly to the instructions he has given them, priority always being given to the best interests of the sportsman's or athlete's health and safety, and not the outcome of the competition.

8  To enable him to carry out his ethical obligations the sports physician must see his authority fully recognized and upheld, particularly wherever it concerns the health, safety and legitimate interests of the sportsman or athlete, none of which can be prejudiced to favour the interests of any third party whatsoever.

9  The sports physician should endeavour to keep the patient's personal physician fully informed of facts relevant to his treatment. If necessary he should collaborate with him to ensure that the sportsman or athlete does not exert himself in ways detrimental to his health and does not use potentially harmful techniques to improve his performance.

10  In sports medicine, as in all other branches of medicine, professional confidentiality must be observed. The right to privacy over medical attention the sportsman or athlete has received must be protected, especially in the case of professional sportsmen or athletes.

11 The sports doctor must not be party to any contract which obliges him to reserve particular forms of therapy solely and exclusively for any one sportsman or athlete or group of sportsmen or athletes.

12 It is desirable that sports physicians from foreign countries, when accompanying a team in another country, should enjoy the right to carry out their specific functions.

13 The participation of a sports physician is desirable when sports regulations are being drawn up.

Following the gross transgression of medical ethics during the Second World War, the World Medical Association (founded largely at the instigation of the BMA) restated the Hippocratic Oath in a modern style, this being known as the *Declaration of Geneva*. Upon this, an *International Code of Medical Ethics* was based.

Whilst these pages were being completed in mid-1997 the British Medical Association was debating at its Annual Meeting the relevance and content of the Oath, in its current form: and the *Sunday Telegraph's* Health correspondent Victoria MacDonald cited (29th June 1997). Dr Irvine Loudon, a medical historian, on the eve of the meeting, said that the present Oath has no relevance today. 'It is daft. People's ethical behaviour is not founded on a ceremonial oath but on those who teach them, their peers and the law of the land.'

## DECLARATION OF GENEVA

At the time of being admitted as a Member of the Medical Profession I solemnly pledge myself to consecrate my life to the service of humanity.

I will give to my teachers the respect and gratitude which is their due;

I will practise my profession with conscience and dignity;

The health of my patient will be my first consideration;

I will respect the secrets which are confided in me;

I will maintain by all the means in my power the honour and the noble traditions of the medical profession;

My colleagues will be my brothers;

I will not permit considerations of religion, nationality, race, party politics or social standing to intervene between my duty and my patient;

I will maintain the utmost respect for human life from the time of conception; even under threat, I will not use my medical knowledge contrary to the laws of humanity.

I make these promises solemnly, freely and upon my honour.

Appendix III

# Reviving ethics in sports
# Time for physicians to act

by Andrew Pipe, MD who is the physician for Canada's National Men's Basketball Team and Chair of the Canadian Centre for Ethics in Sport. In 1992 he served as chief medical officer to Canada's Olympic Team. He practices at the University of Ottawa Heart Institute and is an editorial board member of the *Physician and Sports Medicine.*

'When will we face the fact that we're producing some really ugly, violent young men?' observed my friend, an internationally prominent basketball coach, who is given neither to hand-wringing nor to strident overstatement. His disquieting words cast a pall over an already disheartening conversation about the state of con- temporary sports. The evils and excesses in sports are, indeed, many and serious. And physicians who care for athletes are not just innocent bystanders. We are affected by the problems, and we have a responsibility and opportunity to combat them.

## DISILLUSIONMENT WITH SPORTS

Sports are often glibly described as a way for athletes to develop character and skills for living. Sadly recent sports-related events and the resulting public disillusionment suggest that this may be more myth than reality. In fact, evidence suggests that athletes may have a higher risk for maladaptive behaviors than their nonathletic peers (Nattiv *et al*, 1997).

The public has begun to lose patience with these negative behaviours of athletes and others in sports. Frequent reports of gratuitous violence, bizarre and hazardous training practices, drug use and doping scandals, the emotional, physical, and sexual abuse of young athletes, the charades that can surround college sports, and the mindless behaviour of some professional athletes have left people disenchanted. The bloated salaries of professional athletes have also contributed to public disillusionment. Sports officials, dazzled by sold-out stadiums, huge television contracts, and sycophantic news media, can be particularly oblivious to public disenchantment.

## AN INTERNATIONAL PHENOMENON

Disenchantment has led citizens of many countries to take action. When the Australian national track and field organization was hiring a director for its programmes, it turned to a former East German coach who was linked directly to the systematic administration of performance-enhancing drugs now known to be characteristic of the excesses of that regime. Australians were outraged, and, after a nationwide outcry, the decision was reversed. In the United States, the National Coalition Against Violent Athletes was formed to educate the public about assaults by athletes, provide victims with referrals for legal advice and counselling, and encourage college officials and professional team administrators to punish abusive athletes aggressively (*Sports Illustrated*, March 16, 1998: 20–22).

Confidential polling of Canadians indicates that parents are withholding their children from participation in certain sports because of concerns about institutionalized violence and drug use (Paul Melia, personal communication, July 1996).

French authors have called for the creation of an independent national commission to protect the rights of adolescent athletes. The appeal is accompanied by a plea that physicians and those who supervise training programs respect professional ethical principles and be guaranteed independence to address athletes' training and well-being (Franck and Olagnier, 1996).

## DIVIDED LOYALTIES

As sports medicine physicians, we have unique ethical responsibilities concerning the athletes in our care, the sports organizations we work for, and the ideals of sportsmanship and fair competition. It is easy at times, when caught up in the pressure of competition, to lose sight of the full range of responsibilities. The temptation is to focus only on the individual athlete's capacity to perform, while ignoring the broader implications of the physician–patient relationship or the need for leadership in addressing problems in sports.

Our primary responsibility is to protect athletes' health and well-being as defined most broadly. Superficially this role may seem perfectly compatible with the interest of the sports organization with which we and the athlete are associated. However, what's best for an athlete's long-term health may conflict with the organization's short-term interest in winning. As a result, we may have a problem of divided loyalty which raises significant questions about the ethical practice of our profession.

Furthermore, medical organizations now pay – in cash or kind – for the right to care for some teams or leagues, presumably because of the publicity these groups receive. It is difficult to be anything but suspicious about this kind of arrangement. Are the athletes' best interests being served when the responsibility for their care is awarded to the highest bidder?

This arrangement raises a larger issue as well. Many people in North America have little or no access to medical care. The spectacle of medical organizations lining up to pay for the opportunity to provide such care to athletes fosters cynicism toward sports and medicine. As long as patients are famous, this practice seems to say medical providers will actually pay to capture some of the publicity glow, while the unknown and uninsured must pay the full fare for their care – or do without.

## WHAT CAN WE DO?

Given these trends, what are our responsibilities to athletes, athletic organizations, and the sports world? We must lend our training, experience, and scientific perspective to the identification and resolution of a range of sporting issues.

### Intervene with patients

Physicians who care for high school or community-based athletes can help their patients – and often patients' parents – to place sports aspirations in a realistic perspective. Physicians who care for college athletes can intervene to minimize their identified risk-taking behaviours (Nattiv *et al*, 1997).

### Speak out

We can be credible spokespersons for the elimination of gratuitous violence, the enhancement of safety and the disavowal of harmful training practices and environments. The rate of athletic injury is a significant public health concern in many countries and remains a challenge for sports medicine physicians. We have a particular responsibility to speak out forcefully about rules that compromise health and safety or impose unrealistic demands on athletes or their physicians. Physicians must recognize their special obligation regarding drug use. Antidoping rules should be clear, consistent, scientifically based, and focused on performance-enhancing substances. Sports should feature competition among athletes, not contests among biological preparations.

## Develop a code of ethics

A fundamental step to promote ethical conduct in sports medicine, and in sports generally would be the development of a sports medicine code of ethics. Such a code would illuminate our obligations and identify the tenets of responsible professional practice in the sports arena.

## Sports physicians as stewards

Most of us have continued to be involved in sports because of our own positive experiences. We understand the powerful role of sports in the physical and emotional development of youth and recognize the importance of exercise to the health of the communities we serve.

We also appreciate sports as a potent cultural force that deserves *and requires* thoughtful stewardship. If we engage in that stewardship by helping sports institutions confront broad social issues and by lending our ethical perspective to the resulting debates, we can help create a sports culture that encourages fair competition and truly promotes the well-being of athletes and society.

Address correspondence to Andrew Pipe, MD, University of Ottawa Heart Institute, 1053 Carling Ave, Ottawa, Ontario, Canada K1Y 4E9.

## References

Franck, A. and Olagnier H. (1996) Consentiment et dependence pour l'adolescent sportif de haut-niveau. *Medecine et Hygiene*, **54**, 1393–6.

Nattiv, A, Puffer, J. C. and Green, G. G. (1997) Lifestyles and health risks of collegiate athletes: a multi-center study. *Clin. J. Sport Med.*, **7(4)**, 262–72.

Appendix IV

# British National Formulary[*]:
# Classified Notes on Drugs and Preparations

## DOPING CLASSES AND METHODS OF THE INTERNATIONAL OLYMPIC COMMITTEE MEDICAL COMMISSION 1997.

The following are examples of classes and methods prohibited in sport:

| | |
|---|---|
| Classes | Stimulants, e.g. amphetamine, bromanian, caffeine (above 12 µg/ml), cocaine, ephedrine, certain agonists. |
| | Narcotics, e.g. diamorphine (heroin), morphine, methadone, pethidine. |
| | Anabolic agents, e.g. methanedienone, nandrolone, stenozolol, testosterone, clanbuterol, DHEA. |
| | Diuretics, e.g. acetazolamide, frusemide, hydrochlorothiazide, triamterene. |
| | Peptide and glycoprotein hormones and analogues, e.g. growth hormone, corticotrophin, chorionic gonadotrophin, erythropoietin. |
| Methods | Blood doping. |
| | Pharmacological, chemical and physical manipulation, e.g. substances and methods that alter the integrity and validity of the urine such as protein acid, catheterization, urine substitutes. |
| Classes of drugs subject to certain restrictions | Alcohol and marijuana: restricted in certain sports. Refer to regulations of national or international federations. |
| | Local anaesthetics: route of administration restricted to local or intra-articular injection. |
| | Corticosteroids: route of administration restricted to topical, inhalation, local or intra-articular injection. |
| | Beta-blockers: restricted in certain sports. Refer to regulations of international sports federations. |

Written notification of administration should be given to relevant medical authority, e.g. governing body medical officer.

[*] From Number 35, March 1998. Reproduced with permission from the British Medical Association and the Royal Pharmaceutical Society of Great Britain.

## TREATMENT GUIDELINES

*Examples of permitted and prohibited substances*

|  | ALLOWED | BANNED |
|---|---|---|
| Asthma | Salbutamol*, larbulanine*, salmeterol*, beclomethasone*, fluticasone*, theophylline* (*by inhalation only), sodium cromoglycate. | Products containing sympathomimetics, e.g. ephedrine, isoprenaline, fenoterol, rinniterol, arciprenaline. |
| Cold/cough | Antibiotics, steam and methol inhalations, permitted antihistamines, barienadrine, aslenizole, photcodine, gualphenosin, dextromethorphan, paracetamol. | Products containing sympathomimetics, e.g. ephedrine, pseudoephedrine, phenylpropanolamine. |
| Diarrhoea | Diphenoxylate, loperamide, products containing electrolytes (e.g. Dioralyte, Rehidran). | Products containing opioids (e.g. morphine). |
| Hay fever | Antihistamines, nasal sprays containing a corticosteroid or xylometazoline, eye drops containing sodium cromoglycate. | Products containing ephedrine, pseudoephedrine. |
| Pain | Aspirin, codeine, dihydrocodeine, ibuprofen, paracetamol, all non-steroidal anilinilammazones, dextropropoxyphene. | Products containing opioids, caffeine. |
| Vomiting | Domperidone, metoclopramide. |  |

WARNING. Some vitamin, herbal and nutritional substances may contain prohibited substances, such as Guaranu, Ma Huang, Chinese ephedrine.

The substances listed are only examples of substances permitted or prohibited by the IOC. Not all sports adopt the IOC Medical Code. If in doubt check with your governing body or with the UKSC Drug Information line 0171-380 8030.

Similar cards detailing classes of drugs and doping methods prohibited by the Football Association and the Lawn Tennis Association are also available.

Reproduced with permission from the British Medical Association and the Royal Pharmaceutical Society of Great Britain.

Appendix V

# Selected organizations with a role in sports medicine

Adapted from and with acknowledgements and extensions to Appendix IV in the British Medical Association's Board of Education and Science, 1996, *Sport and Exercise Medicine: Policy and Provision* see page 10 of main text.

## 1. UNITED KINGDOM

### *Association of Chartered Physiotherapists in Sports Medicine (ACPSM)*

81 Heol West Plas
Coity
Bridgend
Glamorgan CF35 6BA
Tel: 01222 735515
Fax: 01222 735821

### *British Association for Sport and Law (BASL)*

School of Law
Elizabeth Gaskell Campus
Hathersage Road
Manchester M13 0JA
Tel: 0161 247 6445
Fax: 0161 247 6309

### *British Association of Sport and Exercise Sciences (BASES)*

The British Association of Sport and Exercise Sciences
114 Cardigan Road
Headingley
Leeds LS6 3BJ
Tel: 0113 231 9606

### British Association of Sport and Medicine (BASM)

BASM
c/o Birch Lee
67 Springfield Lane
Eccleston
St Helens WA10 5HB
Tel/Fax:   01744 28198

### British Olympic Association (BOA)

British Olympic Association
1 Wandsworth Plain
Wandsworth
London SW18 1EH
Tel:   0181 871 2677
Fax: 0181 871 9104

### British Olympic Medical Centre (BOMC)

British Olympic Medical Centre
Northwick Park Hospital
Watford Road
Harrow
Middlesex HA1 3UJ
Tel:   0181 864 0609
Fax: 0181 864 8738

### The British Orthopaedic Sports Trauma Association

The British Orthopaedic Sports Trauma Association
D J Edwards MB FRCS
Secretary to the Society
at the British Orthopaedic Association
Royal College of Surgeons
35–43 Lincoln's Inn Fields
London WC2A 3PN
Tel:   0171 405 6507

### Central Council of Physical Recreation

Francis House
Francis Street
London SW1PE 1DE
Tel:   0171 828 3163
Fax: 0171 630 8820

**Chartered Society of Physiotherapy**

14 Bedford Row
London WC1R 4ED
Tel:  0171 242 1941

**Disability Sport England**

Solecast House
13–27 Brunswick Place
London N1 6DX
Tel/Fax: 0171 490 4919

**The Institute of Sports Medicine**

At University College London Medical School
Charles Bell House
67–73 Riding House Street
London W1P 7LD
Tel/Fax: 0171 813 2832

**Lilleshall Sports Injury and Human Performance Centre**

Lilleshall National Sports Centre
Near Hemport
Shropshire TF10 9AT
Tel:  01952 605028 (Rehabilitation Clinic)
Tel:  01952 670185 (Human Performance Clinic)

**Medical Officers of Schools Association**

Medical Society of London
11 Chandos Street
London W1M 0EB
Tel:  01732 750 586

**National Sports Medicine Institute**

National Sports Medicine Institute of the United Kingdom
c/o Medical College of St Bartholomew's Hospital
Charterhouse Square
London EC1M 6BQ
Tel:  0171 251 0583
Fax: 0171 251 0774

## Royal Society of Medicine

Section of Sports Medicine
Royal Society of Medicine
1A Wimpole Street
London W1M 8AE
Tel: 0171 290 2987
Fax: 0171 290 2989

## Scottish Institute of Sports Medicine and Sports Science

University of Strathclyde
Jordanhill Campus
76 Southbrac Drive
Glasgow G13 1PP
Tel: 0141 950 3189
Fax: 0141 950 3175

## Scottish Sports Council

Caledonian House
South Gyle
Edinburgh EH12 9DQ
Tel: 0131 317 7200
Fax: 0131 317 7202

## Special Olympics UK

The Otis Building
43–59 Clapham Road
London SW9 0JI

## Sports Committee of the Medical Commission on Accident Prevention

Professor J. E. Davies
Chairman
The Medical Commission on Accident Prevention
35–43 Lincoln's Inn Fields
London WC2A 3PN
Tel/Fax: 0171 242 3176

## Sports Council for Northern Ireland

House of Sport
Upper Malone Road
Belfast BT9 5LA
Tel: 01232 381 222
Fax: 01232 686 757

**Sports Council for Wales**

Welsh Institute of Sports
Sophia Gardens
Cardiff CF1 9SW
Tel:  01222 300 500
Fax: 01222 300 600

**Sport England** (formerly the English Sports Council)

16 Upper Woburn Place
London WC1H 0QP
Tel:  0171 273 1500
Fax: 0171 383 5740

**UK Sports Council**

Walkden House
3–10 Melton Street
London NW1 2EB
Tel:  0171 380 8000
Fax: 0171 380 8010

**Youth Sport Trust**

Rutland Hall
Loughborough University
Loughborough
Leicestershire LE11 3TU
Tel:  01509 228293
Fax: 01509 210851

## 2. OVERSEAS

**American Academy of Podiatric Sports Medicine (AAPSM)**

1729 Glastonberry Road
Potomac, MD 20854
USA
Tel:  00 1 800 438 3355

### American Academy of Sports Physicians (AASP)

c/o Geriatric Research Education Center
VA Medical Center
University of Florida
1601 Archer Road
Gainesville, FL 32608
USA
Tel:  00 1 904 374 6077
Fax: 00 1 904 335 1360

### American College of Sports Medicine (ACSM)

Box 1440
Indianapolis, IN 46206-1440
USA
Tel: 00 1 317 637 9200

### American Medical Society for Sports Medicine (AMSSM)

7611 Elmwood Avenue
Suite 202
Middleton, WI 53562
USA

### Australian Sports Medicine Federation

PO Box 897
Belconnen, ACT 2616
Australia
Tel:  00 61 6 251 6944
Fax: 00 61 6 253 1489

### Canadian Academy of Sports Medicine and the Sports Medicine Council of Canada (CASM)

1600 James Naismith Drive
Suite 502
Gloucester, ON K1B 5N4
Canada
Tel:  00 1 613 748 5851

### Canadian Association for Health, Physical Education, Recreation and Dance (CAHPERD)

Place R Tait McKenzie
1600 James Naismith Drive
Gloucester, ON K1B 5N4
Canada
Tel:  00 1 613 748 5622

**European Federation of Sports Medicine**
Professor G Giovdano-Lanza
President
Urf de Medecine
rue Léonard de Vinci 74
F-93012, Bobigny Cedex
France
Tel:  00 33 1 4838 7613
Fax: 00 33 1 4838 7777

**Fédération Internationale de Médicine Sportive (FIMS)**
Professor Dr Eduardo de Rose
General Secretary
c/o Dr Albert Dirix
J de Pauwstraat 35
SINT NIKLAS
9100 Belgium
Tel:  00 32 3776 0089

**International Council of Sports Science and Physical Education**
Am Kleinen Wannsee 6
14109 Berlin
Germany
Tel:  00 49 30 80 500 360
Fax: 00 49 30 563 86

**International Medical Society of Paraplegia**
National Spinal Injury Centre
Stoke Mandeville Hospital
Aylesbury
Bucks, HP21 8AL
UK

**International Olympic Committee**
Chateau de Vidy
1007 Lausanne
Switzerland
Tel:  00 41 21 621 61 11
Fax  00 41 21 621 62 16
Website: http://www.olympic.org

**International Paralympic Committee**
Residentie Lodewojk 1
Abdijbekestraat 4B bus 6
8200 Bruge
Belgium
Tel:  00 32 50 38 93 40
Fax: 00 32 50 39 01 19

**International School Sport Federation**
Postfach 65
1014 Vienna
Austria

**International Sports Organisation for the Disabled**
Newmarket
Ontario L3Y 2K2
Canada

**International Stoke Mandeville Wheelchair Sports Federation**
ISMWSF Secretariat
Olympic Village
Barnard Crescent
Aylesbury
Bucks, HP21 9PP
Tel:  00 44 1296 436179
Fax: 00 44 1296 436484

**Sports Science Institute of South Africa**
Boundary Road
Newlands 7700
Cape Town
South Africa

**The World Medical Association, Inc.**
28 avenue des Alpes
BP 63-01212 Ferney-Voltaire Cedex
France
Tel:  00 33 4 50 40 75 75
Fax: 00 33 4 50 40 59 37

# List of Cases

Affuto-Nartoy v Clark and ILEA (1984) *The Times*, 9 February, 62, 67, 72

Airedale NHS Trust v Bland [1993] 1 All ER 821, 93

Alcock v Chief Constable of South Yorkshire Police [1991] 4 All ER 907, 130

Attorney General v Hastings Corporation (1950) 94 Sol Jo 225, 127

Bacon v White (1998) *New Law Digest*, 14 June, 79

Baker v Jones (1954) I A.E.R. 533, 25

Baker v Kaye (1996) *The Times*, 13 December, [1997] IRLR 214, 106, 107

Ballard v North British Railway Co (1923) SC (HL) 43 at 46, 39

Barfoot v East Sussex CC (1930) (unreported: *The Head's Legal Guide*, para 3-iii [Croner Publications], 70

Barkway v South Wales Transport Co Ltd [1950] 1 All ER 398 at 399, 39

Beaumont v Surrey CC (1968) 66 LGR 580, 112 SJ 704, 71

Benitez v New York City Board of Education (1989) 541 NE 2d, NY Ct App, 104

Bidwell v Parks (1982) (unreported), 55

Bolam v Friern Barnet Hospital Management Committee [1957] 1 WLR 582 at 587, 2 All ER 188, 27, 35

Bolitho v City and Hackney H.A. [1997] 4 AER 771, 27, 35

Bolton v Stone [1951] AC 850, 127

Britton v Bradford City Association Football Club and others (1987) *Times, Daily Telegraph*, 24 February, 130

Brown v Lewis (1896) 12 TLR 455, 38, 129

Cameron Sharp v North Cumbria Health Authority (1997) *Daily Telegraph*, 18 February, (1997) *Guardian*, 20 February, 94

Casey Martin v US PGA (1998), Weiler Roberts: *Sports and the Law* 2nd edn, 93

Cassidy v Ministry of Health [1951] 2 KB 343 at 365, [1951] 1 All ER 574 at 588, 39

Castle v St Augustine's Links Ltd (1922) 38 TLR 615, 127

Higgins v North West Metropolitan Regional Hospital Board (1955) 1 All ER, 31
Hilder v Associated Portland Cement Manufacturers [1961] 1 WLR 1434, 127
Hundely v Rite Aid and Jones, [South Carolina], 90
Hunter v Hanley [1955] SLT 213 and 217, 35

Jones v WRU (1997) *Times*, 6 March, 25

Kapfunde v Abbey National and Anor (1988) CAT 98-0495, 107
Keating v Tottenham Hotspur (1997) *Times*, 17 July, 94
Kennaway v Thompson [1980] 3 All ER 329, 128
Knapp v Northwestern University (1996) No. 96-3450, US Ct of App 7th Cir, 22 November, 93

La Fleur v Cornelis (1979) 28 NBR (2d) 569 NBSC, 29–30
Lacey v Parker and Boyle (for Jordans CC) (1994) 144 NLJ 785, 128
Lamond v Glasgow Corporation (1968) SLT 291, 55, 127–8
Langham v Governors of Wellingborough School and Fryer (1932) 101 LKJB 513, 147 LT 91; 96 JP 236; 30 LGR 276, 69
Larkin v Archdiocese of Cincinnati (1990) No. C-1-90-619, SD OHIO, 31 August, 92–3
Lucille Gathers *et al* v Loyola Marymount *et al*, [M. J. Greenberg], 77

McCord v Swansea City High Court London (1996), 57
MacDonald v York County Hospital Corporation [1972] 28 DLR 3d 521, 40, 94
Martin M Krimsky, Administrator for Estate of Eric Wilson Gathers, Jr, and Michael Horsey, Guardian of the Estate of Aaron Kevin Crump v Loyola Marymount University *et al* [M. J. Greenberg], 77
May v Strong (1990) (Halsbury's Laws MRE 92/62) All Eng AR (1991), 56
Maynard v West Midlands Regional Health Authority [1985] 1 All ER 635, [1984] 1 WLR 634, 35
Miller v Jackson [1977] 1 QB 966, 128
Modahl v British Athletic Federation (1995), *New Law Journal* Vol. 145: 20 January, 63
Mogabgab v Orleans Parish School Board (1970) 239 So 2d 456, 103
Moore v Hampshire CC (1981) 80 LGR 481, 71
Morrell v Owen (1993) *Times*, 14 December, 63, 72

# Index

# Sport and the Law
Third edition

## Edward Grayson, MA (Oxon)
*Barrister of the Middle Temple and of the South-Eastern Circuit; Visiting Professor of Sport and the Law in the Anglia Law School, Anglia Polytechnic University; Founding President, British Association for Sport and Law; Fellow of the Royal Society of Medicine.*

**It only takes a second to score a goal ...**

*"It is rare to find a textbook as readable as this ... a book from which anyone advising or connected with the running of a sports club cannot fail to benefit."*
**Law Society's Gazette (Review of second edition)**

The third edition of this classic text within 10 years brings the reader fully up to date with the increasing number of legal issues arising from sport. It enables the reader to understand the importance of key cases, and relevant legislation.

It covers every aspect of the subject: from major sporting events and violence to agents, contracts and taxation; from disciplinary tribunals to grass roots problems at school, club, and village green levels; to sponsorship of this great slice of the international commercial entertainment branch of the sprawling leisure industry.

It is a timeless and topical text for all sports law litigators and anyone involved in running a sports club or organization, in this daily exploding area of health, education, and the Rule of Law throughout the world.

Publication date: September 1999
ISBN: 0 406 90505 3
Product code: GSL3
Pre-publishing price: Approximately £48.00

Order by telephone to Butterworths' Customer Services Department
Telephone: 0181 662 2000; Fax: 0181 662 2012